The
Herbal Way to
Natural Health
and Beauty

Other titles of similar interest from
Random House Value Publishing, Inc.:

A-Z Guide to Herbal Remedies
Alternative Healing Secrets
Ancient Healing Secrets
Art of Aromatherapy
Growing and Using Healing Herbs
The Healing Benefits of Garlic
Herbal Home Companion
Herbal Medicine
Herbal Tonic Therapies
Herbs: Their Culture and Uses
Massage and Aromatherapy
Natural Healing Secrets
World of Herbs

The
Herbal Way to
Natural Health
and Beauty

Dian Dincin Buchman

GRAMERCY BOOKS

New York

In loving memory of my parents
Renee Dincin and Herman Dincin

Copyright © 1973, 1995 by Dian Dincin Buchman

This 2000 edition is published by Gramercy Books™, an imprint of Random House Value Publishing, Inc. 201 East 50th Street, New York, N.Y. 10022 by arrangement with NTC/Contemporary Group, Chicago, Ill.

Gramercy Books™ and design are trademarks of Random House Value Publishing, Inc.

Printed and bound in the United States of America.

(Originally published as: *The Complete Herbal Guide to Natural Health and Beauty*)

Random House
New York • Toronto • London • Sydney • Auckland
http://www.randomhouse.com/

Library of Congress Cataloging–in–Publication Data

Buchman, Dian Dincin.
    [Complete herbal guide to natural health and beauty]
  The herbal way to natural health and beauty / Dian Dincin Buchman.
        p. cm.
    Originally published: The complete herbal guide to natural health and beauty. New Canaan, Conn. : Keats Pub. Co.,Inc., 1973.
    Includes index.
    ISBN 0-517-20711-7
    1. Herbs--Therapeutic use. 2. Herbal cosmetics. I. Title.

RM666.H33 B83 2000
615'.321—dc21   99-046514

8 7 6 5 4 3 2 1

The Herbal Way to Natural Healthy and Beauty is not intended as medical advice. Its intent is solely informational and educational. Please consult a health professional should the need for one be indicated.

CONTENTS

ACKNOWLEDGMENTS

For invaluable help in research and preparation for this book I have to thank Alexander Dubenchiek, who kept me informed on the chemistry of the herbs. Ira Kapp, president of Felton International, generously supplied me with most of the oils, perfumes and materials for making lotions and creams. The late Elizabeth Hall, senior librarian of the Horticultural Society of New York; Julia Weiss of the Mahopac Library and Mid-Hudson System; specialists, and rare book librarians at the New York Academy of Medicine; and Dorothy Gomez of the Royal Horticultural Society of London were all helpful in the research. The late Vivian Heisler lovingly shared her time, wit and intelligence.

Finally my deepest dept is due to three: my grandmother Anna-Pearl whose knowledge of herbal lore started me in my lifelong pursuit; and her daughter, my mother, Renee Dincin, and especially my father Herman Dincin, whose unquenching curiosity about natural medicine and cures lit within me a need to investigate and experiment with remedies and cures from many cultures.

Preparing the revision of this work brought up memories of its genesis—the summer I was seven, and much later, the summer of '69.

The year I am seven the Dincin clan is temporarily low in funds, so at vacation time, Dad persuades a friend to rent us his run-down barn. Amazingly, it is only a short walk from a pristine lake. My father starts a Herculean battle to rid the barn of its bats, mice, and snakes. Later as I watch, he gets the artesian hand pump going, and improvises an indoor camp-style kitchen. Meanwhile Mom cleans the outhouse with whitewash and herbal antiseptics.

This great adventure is made all the more magical by the arrival of my grandmother, who takes us daily through fields and woods where she painstakingly collects roots, flowers, leaves, berries, even (cherry) bark, which she needs to make her favorite preparations.

In that make-do kitchen my grandmother produces any number of tonics, liniments, lotions, syrups, medicines and beauty products. One day there is the unforgettable miracle of her cold cream. First rose water, then lanolin and melted beeswax and Grandma has her cleansing cream. Another time she adds just-picked-berries, and the barn is permeated with the heavenly smell of strawberries.

I learn the secrets of my grandmother's peaches-and-cream skin; and by watching and listening I learn how some plants can gently prevent and remedy a variety of problems. *That summer was the invisible launching of my herbal knowledge and curiosity.*

Jump to the hot summer of 1969. It is a summer with many highs and lows. The low is the Vietnam war quagmire—the highs include enjoying the good life in a cottage on a seven-mile lake;

and the unforgettable exhilaration of Neil Armstrong's walk on the moon.

This is the year I somehow rediscover my grandmother's nostrums. This happens because I am disenchanted with synthetic drugs and the overuse of antibiotics. I have been made aware of the chemicals and pesticides in my environment and I am beginning to distrust the use of hormones in our poultry and meat products. I want more control over my own health destiny, and I want to be more connected to nature. I investigate my family lore.

A few weeks prior to the moonwalk, an old pal, Michael, drops over to say hello to us. In his role as Extension Director of a nearby university he asks me to create a "cutting-edge" course in non-drug health remedies. I jump at the chance and call it *The Dynamics of Wholistic Good Health.* Note the spelling. In '69 we didn't know if we should call it Wholistic or holistic. As I work out herbal experiments and varied details for the course—the day of the moonwalk—a lightbulb flashes in my head. *Should I do a book on my old family recipes?* Can I assemble a herbal beauty guide?

It is the oddest confluence of past and future. The very day the USA proves it can conquer space, I choose to delve deeper into the "useful" past. That same day, I have another thought. I suddenly realize I must include *nutrition* in my herbal book! I have been quietly studying nutrition for several years and somehow I am in the vanguard with the then limited group of people who understand the connection between nutrition and good health. Now as I look back some 25 years later it seems unbelievable to recall how friends, including many doctors, laughed disdainfully if one mentioned the correlation of vitamins and health. The nicest remark at that time is "It can't hurt, I suppose." Nevertheless, I decide to include whatever is known about the impact of vitamins and minerals on good looks.

I start to research and verify old family recipes. To expand my personal repertoire, I pore over hundreds of rare old "receipt" books, old herbals, fascinating handwritten and personal journals of bygone women, often famous beauties. I collect wonderful and useful material. I spend time in medical and rare-book libraries in

New York, Washington and especially in London where plant medicine is actively practiced by well-trained herbalists.

The book enjoyed a highly gratifying success, not only in this country but in England, Scotland, Wales, Ireland, Australia and New Zealand, and over the years I had many letters of interest from readers. One of my favorite memories is a correspondence with a delightful New Zealander who complains that while she is not that old, her fragile Celtic skin plus the sun has made her neck look wretchedly ancient. Can I help her design a regimen to restore her neck? I point out the parts of the book which she can use—the things that can soften skin crinkles. She soon writes to tell me she is looking better and going on a cruise. Months later I receive a charming note saying she is to be married to an English nobleman whom she met on that cruise. I am astonished when she says it wouldn't have been possible without my help!

What has happened in the intervening years since I conceived this book? Why, herbs and plants for medicine have come into their own once again. Scientific research in many journals repeatedly verifies ancient herbal remedies, among them ginger for nausea and motion sickness, garlic for some heart problems and hypertension, cranberry juice for cystitis and acidophilus yogurt for yeast infections.

Recently *The New York Times* ran a feature from Paris, "So It's Not What Doctor Ordered. Herbs Are In," describing a return to the use of plants in France.*

Botany has virtually disappeared from the curriculum of France's medicine and pharmacy students, and the country's mighty pharmaceutical industry has moved ever deeper into synthetic drugs and biotechnology.

Yet more and more French men and women, tens of thousands of them, are taking herbs. The French . . . these days are turning again to grandmother's old herbal concoctions to help their digestion, sleep, jangled nerves and abused livers.

Herbal medicine is only part of the country's growing movement toward a less high-tech approach to treating the sick. As

*New York Times, International Section, April 11, 1994, Marlise Simon

in other European countries, there is a rising interest in France in alternative and preventive medicine.

In Paris, a recent survey found that one in five households now uses herbal remedies. Even at elegant Parisian dinner tables, chances are that an "infusion" appears of verbena, linden or mint to dispatch a meal.

The same renewal of interest in herbs for beauty and health has occurred in other European countries, and in America. This change in interest in alternative and herbal medicine is confirmed in a survey in the prestigious *New England Journal of Medicine*.* In response to the survey, the director of the Office of Alternative Medicine tells *The New York Times* "the popularity of alternative medicine demonstrates a hunger among Americans for a more humane and less invasive type of treatment than that ordinarily practiced by standard doctors."†

The study, conducted by Dr. David M. Eisenberg of Beth Israel Hospital and Harvard Medical School in Boston, found that Americans spent a whopping $13.7 million on alternative medicine in 1990, most of it not reimbursed by insurance.

When I conceived this book, there were all too few herbal resources. Now I am able to supply you with many excellent local and mail order services throughout the country. A surprising number of mail order resources offer toll-free 800 numbers. Today there are many national and international holistic organizations throughout the world you can contact for information. In this edition, in addition to herbal information on tea tree oil, echinacea and gingko, I provide many new nutritional support and other charts for sleep, the eyes, hair, nails, and skin, including the dos and don'ts of tanning, and the sun and skin cancer.

DIAN DINCIN BUCHMAN
New York

New England Journal of Medicine, January 28, 1993
†*New York Times,* January 28, 1993, Natalie Angier

CHAPTER I

HOW TO USE HERBS

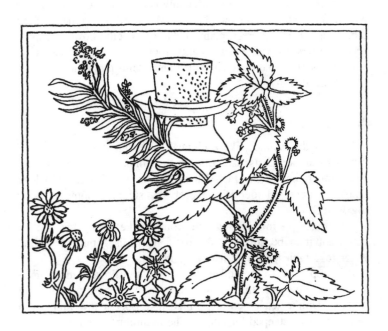

Some people can/Some people can't/Tell the difference between/
Gary Cooper and Cary Grant./

This little humorous verse somehow reminds me of the erb-herb
controversy and the disparity in British and American pronunciation. For some obscure reason we Americans call herbs "erb,"
dropping the *h* as if we were Cockneys from the play *Pygmalion*.
However, we usually refer to books on this subject as herbal, and

call the practitioners of the herbal craft herbalists, pronouncing the *h*'s in all these words.

I often go back and forth between the United States and Great Britain and I sometimes feel like a schizophrenic trying to adapt to each country's preferred pronunciation. I am therefore starting a one-woman movement to unite these two pronunciations into one. *H* for all these words, please.

Then there is a question of what any book called a herbal should and could include. Over the centuries the word has come to mean almost any growing green plant, including specific flowers, leaves, seeds, berries, as well as such barks, roots, tree sap, grasses, fungi and even shrubs that have cherished and useful properties for food or botanic therapy.

Infusion

Perhaps this sounds like a clinical term, but it is the word all professional herbalists use. But do not think of it in laboratory terms but rather of the fact that all leaves and flowers will lend you their personal identities merely by steeping some in boiling water.

You make an infusion as you would make strong tea. Unless you want it to be stronger, the basic recipe is 1 pint of boiling water to 2 tablespoons of leaves or flowers.

It is important to remember that leaves and flowers must *never be boiled.* You pour the boiling water *over* the herb, and you let it steep. Unlike tea or coffee, which take only a few minutes, a herb should be steeped far longer. The minimum time for cosmetic use (it takes longer for medicinal use) is 15 minutes, but the longer you allow the herb to steep the stronger and more valuable it becomes. Three hours is the maximum time needed to extract the properties fully.

Always keep the pot covered during steeping. After steeping, herbs will fall to the bottom of the pot; so you can either skim off the water, which is now infused with herb principles, or strain it into a jug.

Use only crockery, glass or ceramic pots, or stainless steel or unbroken enamel-lined pans. *Never use aluminium* or *Teflon* pans to steep a herb. For a sage rinse, if you want it to be darker, you may use an iron pan.

Though it is best to take about 3 hours to release the properties of a herb, often you won't have that much time. You can use a stainless steel teaspoon, or tea holder, which makes enough for 1 cup. Adjust the recipe accordingly.

Another shortcut is to use a coffee infuser. These are made of glass and hold enough for 1 cup. Place 1 or 2 tablespoons of the dried herb in the infuser and pour a cup of boiling water over it. Leave for 3 minutes.

Alternatively, if the herb can be used with milk (as in many facials), *cold* milk absorbs the essences of most herbs *without* heat. Allow 1 tablespoon of the herb to every cup of cold milk. Steep for several hours. Keep the jar covered with a cloth.

Decoction

Decoction is simply boiling. Barks, roots, seeds and chips take at least ½ hour's boiling to release their properties. As with infusions, use stainless steel, crockery or glass only, and remember *to cover the pan* while boiling so as to retain all chemicals and principles released.

Essence

To make an essence, buy an ounce of an essential oil and dissolve it in 1 pint of vodka, gin or brandy, or 70% ethyl alcohol.*

Tincture

Many herbs do not release their properties in water but become active in alcohol (or vinegar). Add 1 ounce of the powdered or crushed herb to 12 ounces† of alcohol, and 4 ounces of water,

*Use ethyl alcohol for *external* tinctures (liniments, perfumes, floral waters, etc.). For *internal* tinctures or tonics use high-grade drinking alcohol such as vodka, gin or brandy. Sherry is sometimes useful too.

†Liquid quantities in ounces are fluid ounces. Buy a fluid ounce cup or jug which makes measuring much easier.

WAYS OF USING DRIED HERBS

	Kind of Herb	Amount	Liquid
Infusion	most leaves, flowers, herbs use cut instead of powdered	2 tablespoons dried herb	1 pint *boiling* water poured over herb and allowed to steep
Short-cut infusion	most leaves, flowers, herbs	1 tablespoon with *stainless steel* tea ball or spoon	1 cup *boiling* water
Milk infusion	most leaves, flowers, herbs	1 tablespoon	1 cup cold milk will absorb essence of herb when impossible to use heat
Decoction	bark, chips, roots, seeds	2 tablespoons (will expand considerably)	boil herb gently in 1 pint or more water
Essence (use externally only)	oil from herb	1 ounce	dissolve in 1 pint alcohol
Tincture	any powdered or crushed herb	1 ounce	12 ounces alcohol
Extraction	any herb, specially aromatic herb	(1) add as much of herb as will fill ½ cup alcohol without crowding; steep 1 week; strain (2) again add leaves and repeat process	ethanol alcohol
Essential oil	aromatic flowers or leaves	2 tablespoons	oil—either corn, olive, or safflower

WAYS OF USING DRIED HERBS (continued)

Container	Minimum Steeping Time	For Best Results
stainless steel, ceramic, glass; never use Teflon or aluminum; iron okay with sage rinse	leave 3 minutes on heat to 15 minutes off heat; cover pot	3 hours away from heat; cover pot
same as infusion; OR French-style coffee infuser, which strains off liquid after water absorbs active principles of herb	3 to 5 minutes	
same as infusion	several hours while covered with porous cloth	
same as infusion	20 minutes cover pot	3 hours cover pot
		store in dark place
tight-lidded jar	stand in full sunlight or warm place for 2 weeks	optional—add 1 teaspoon glycerine—store in dark closet
large tight-lidded jar	(1) soak 1 week; pour off leaves; strain through nylon or cheesecloth (2) again add leaves for 1 week and repeat process	extract is finished when alcohol has characteristic smell of herb. For long-lasting extract add: ¼ tsp. tincture of benzoin, ¼ tsp. boric acid powder dissolved in 3 tbsp. witch hazel; optional extra ½ tsp. peppermint extract
½ pint bottle filled ¾ full with oil and pounded aromatic herb	3 weeks	closed bottle in full sunlight. Every 7 days strain herbs to obtain clear oil; add fresh pounded herbs; oil is ready when it has strong scent

and place in a tight-lidded jar. Let it stand for 2 weeks either in full sunlight (preferably) or in a warm place, or add a teaspoon of glycerine. Store in a dark cupboard.

Herb Extracts

Infusions and decoctions will not last more than a few days outside of a refrigerator. Herb extracts are longer-lasting. For a herbal skin astringent that uses alcohol:

Use a pint jar. To a ½ cup 70% ethyl alcohol or a ½ cup vodka, gin or brandy, add as much of a herb as will fill the jar without crowding. Steep for a week and strain. Add more leaves and repeat the same process. After a week pour off the liquid through a nylon or cheesecloth strainer. The extract is finished when the alcohol retains the characteristic smell of the herb.

To make this extract last longer add: ¼ teaspoon simple tincture of benzoin, ¼ teaspoon boric acid powder, each of these dissolved in 3 tablespoons of witch hazel. If you wish the extract to have a stronger tingling quality add ½ teaspoon of peppermint extract. Use a tightly lidded jar.

CHAPTER II

SKIN

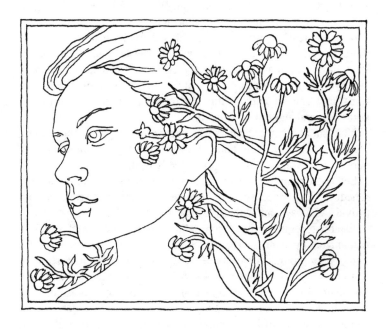

Your skin is one of the miracles of nature, and its perfection should be cherished. It regulates your body temperature, protects you from bacterial invasion and helps you eliminate toxins. If you want your skin to look attractive and healthy, there are several rules you must follow. The most important is cleansing with natural and reviving substances, for a clean skin is bound to look healthier. Since constant washing removes most natural oils and moisture, and even the protective acid covering, you must consciously replace these oils, moisture and acid.

Other factors are diet, sleep, exercise and elimination.

For a radiant skin, drink at least 6 to 8 glasses of pure water a day and eat a diet high in fiber, green and yellow vegetables, fruit, carbohydrates and some protein—a range that includes every vitamin. If the skin needs extra help, two vitamins are indispensable: vitamin A to help in maintenance of the skin, and vitamin E to bolster the function of the skin. E is vital for two reasons: it helps to ward off infections, and it acts like a scavenger of free flowing radical electrons and prevents them from damaging both the skin and the entire immune system. The herb aloe vera has at least three important functions for skin health: it acts as a mild laxative (clears away impurities and helps to overcome constipation), and can be applied directly to the skin to heal sores and abrasions and fight skin infections.

You should get enough sleep each night to wake up feeling completely rested. The amount of sleep varies from person to person. Everyone knows his own needs best.

Set up a routine of body and facial exercises to fit your time schedule. You need such movement to increase circulation and provide your system with additional oxygen.

Establish regular elimination habits, the importance of which is recognized by many herbalists. Retained toxins can show in fatigue, poor color, circles under the eyes or skin blemishes. A couple of figs or prunes a day can help in daily elimination. An excellent aid for chronic constipation is an early morning *cold* drink of lemon juice and water, or a tablespoon of cider vinegar and a tablespoon of honey stirred into a cup of hot or cool water. However, don't be alarmed if your elimination pattern is not a daily one. The best medical opinion is that each person can establish his own natural pattern.

Other factors which influence your looks are tension, overwork and the outside influences of polluted air, overheated offices and homes, and foods riddled with pesticides and depleted of nutrition.

This chapter is devoted to nutritional aids, cleansing methods, herbal and food solutions to skin problems, and techniques for prevention and eradication of blemishes. A word first about who can use what substance on what kind of skin. People with normal skins (are there any?) may use *any* facial complexion water, soap or wrinkle chaser mentioned in this book. But anyone with oily skin, dry skin, large pores, thread veins or facial and body spot problems should use only those food substances, pharmaceuticals or herbs which are specified in pages dealing with these problems. This chapter also gives herbal and nutritional advice on sunbathing, herbal astringents, cosmetic vinegars and deodorants. Chapter III is devoted to all kinds of baths to restore body moisture, tone and softness. For herbal aids to induce sleep—fatigue being a prime contributor to aging skin—see Chapter IX.

You will note many references to lanolin in this chapter, indeed in the whole book. Lanolin is the oil washed from the wool of sheep, which resembles our own skin oil, sebum. It is the perfect moisturizer, being not only an emollient but also a humectant (water retainer). There are two kinds of lanolin, hydrous and anhydrous; in this book I always use *anhydrous* lanolin, i.e., lanolin prepared without water, which acts as a better moisturizer, since it can attract water from the air as well as from the deeper levels of the skin. Always ask for *anhydrous* lanolin when buying it. Some people may be sensitive to lanolin, even in its more purified form. Test its use on a small area of the arm before using it.

1. FACIAL EXERCISES

Try not to tense up your facial muscles when you talk and think, and train yourself to relax your face thoroughly whenever you can. Very often you will discover you are keeping certain muscles in a state of constant tension, particularly the muscles around the mouth. Some people clench or grind their teeth when they are asleep. Once you are aware of this or other grimacing habits, you can consciously change them by suddenly relaxing the tensed muscles completely. Do this every time you become aware of the tension, and soon the relaxed state will be natural to you.

You can do the following exercises anywhere—while doing housework, or even while driving (all except the last two). Anti-wrinkle and antitension exercises are more effective if you first pat a moisturizing cream onto the face, and if you reverse gravity by lying with your head lower than your feet. Lie with your palms facing upward.

There are four ways to achieve this reversal of gravity. One, of course, is the shoulder stand, the other the unique yoga head-stand—but many people find it difficult to maintain either of these stands. A simple way is to lie with your back on the floor with your feet resting on a bed or sofa. The very best and most relaxing and scientific method of reversal is with a *slant board.** A folding, cushioned slant board will help you to lie with your head low, and your feet in the air at just the proper angle. Slant boards are an invaluable beauty aid. Whether you take a facial everyday or not, spend at least 15 minutes a day, preferably at the end of the day, on a slant board, for by reversing normal gravity you will tone and re-energize your body and stimulate blood circulation, particularly on your face, which gets very little exercise.

Open your eyes wide and stare to the count of six.

Contract your nose as if you are sneezing and flare out the nostrils.

Lift the side of your mouth to the right as if you were sneering.

Lift the side of your mouth to the left in the same way.

Open the mouth by keeping the upper lip taut and lower lip down.

Purse your lips together as if to whistle.

Open your mouth as if you were going to shout.

Slowly blow up your cheeks and entire upper and lower mouth area and fill with air. Retain air for a count of fifteen and expel with a quick "plop" sound. This gentle exercise will not only help to avoid laugh-line wrinkles, but if done several times a day, might gradually soften existing lines.

With your fists, iron your forehead slowly from the middle in an upward sweep to the temples.

With the backs of your outstretched fingers, massage your

*Slant boards can be purchased in health food stores, sporting goods or department stores.

chin from the center toward the ear in a medium-strong patting motion.

For a good double-chin exercise, see Section 11.

2. CLEANSING THE SKIN

You cannot look good unless your face is absolutely clean. The frequency of cleansing should depend on the amount of surface dirt acquired as well as on the oiliness of the skin. Those with an oily skin must clean their face of surface dirt more frequently, as they are more apt to develop blemishes.

There are various methods of cleansing the skin. The first I will mention is steaming, since it can deep-clean the pores. It can be used every day by those with normal and oily skin, and once every 2 weeks by those with dry skin. Other cleansing creams, herbal waters, food scrubs and natural soaps can be used once a day by those with dry skin, and several times a day by those with oily or normal skin or as specifically indicated.

Whenever possible, allow the face to breathe at night, free of oils and creams. In this way, various accumulated body toxins will be excreted.

Steaming

Many professionals start a deep cleansing of the face with steaming to open the pores and rid the skin of its impurities. Steam has many uses: it cleanses the skin of surface dirt, stimulates the skin and the circulation, and encourages perspiration, thus helping to get rid of toxins and prevent pimples. For home use I recommend using a simple steam technique or steam combined with a herb infusion. Those with delicate, sensitive skin or those with broken veins on their face *must not use* this technique.

The best face-steaming method with herbs is the foolproof and simple one of pouring boiling water over complexion herbs, improvising a towel-tent, and allowing the steam to soak your face for 10 minutes or more. If you prefer occasionally to use a room vaporizer containing a herb infusion you may do so. But be careful with directed steam from the vaporizer. In cool or cold climates, don't go outside for at least one hour after you have opened your pores in this manner. Once the pores are cleansed, close them by patting with cool water or an astringent such as witch hazel extract.

Different herbs have different properties. Some aid in the cleansing process, some increase circulation, others remove impurities, still others are wrinkle-preventers. A few have the capacity to heal rough skin and lesions. Others tighten and stimulate. Some of these herbs also prevent and control blemishes.

The following herbs can be used for steaming, individually or in combination. Note that these same herbs can be used in facials (see Section 4).

Versatile

chamomile
elder flower

Cleansing, neutral, soothing

chamomile (also good with
    thyme and lavender)

Remove impurities

fennel
nettle
lime flowers (linden)
hay flower extract
oat flowers

Drying/astringent

yarrow
lady's mantle
witch hazel extract

Cleansing/circulation boosters

nettle
rosemary

Stimulating/tightening

peppermint
elder flower
simple tincture of benzoin
balsam of Gilead
gum tragacanth
gum arabic
horsetail

Healing

houseleek
comfrey
fennel

For specific blemish prevention herbs see Section 5.

How to Remove Blackheads after Steaming

You can remove most blackheads and whiteheads after plain or herbal steaming by pushing gently with a tissue or a cotton swab in a gently rotating circle. You will make your task easier by using a makeup mirror with side lights. For the really difficult-to-remove blackheads and whiteheads or other blemishes, see Section 5.

Once you have removed the whiteheads or blackheads, close your pores with such astringents as chamomile or lady's mantle infusion, or peeled cucumber, lemon juice and water, rose water or witch hazel extract. There is a full description of food and herbal astringents in Section 13. If you have no astringents immediately available use cool water, or in the case of normal or oily skin, a piece of ice. However, those with thin skin or thread veins must never subject their skin to extreme temperatures.

Cleansing Cream

Cleansing cream is one of the oldest complexion-care products. It was developed nearly two thousand years ago by the Greek physician Galen, who combined olive oil, wax and rose water. My version is a variation with sweet almond oil (or avocado oil). This is a simple recipe with the purest ingredients; it costs very little and is the equivalent of the most expensive cream on the market.

white wax	½ ounce
anhydrous lanolin	1 ounce
sweet almond oil (or avocado)	3 ounces
rose water	1 ounce

Melt the white wax and lanolin in a double boiler. Slowly add the almond oil and blend in the rose water, stirring all the time. Remove from the heat. Add aromatic oil or essence (optional). Pour into labeled opaque jar.

Cocoa butter is another exceptional cleanser for the skin. Not only is it nourishing for the face, neck and hands, but it has a delightful smell.

You can make a cocoa butter cleansing liquid as follows:

cocoa butter	1 tablespoon
anhydrous lanolin	1 tablespoon
avocado oil (or sweet almond oil or safflower oil)	½ cup

In the top of a double boiler, melt together the cocoa butter, the lanolin and avocado oil until they are all completely dissolved and blended together. Beat with an electric mixer until the combination is slightly cooled. Pour into labeled jar. Shake before using.

To adapt this recipe for dry skin, to every 3 tablespoons of the cocoa butter cleansing liquid, add 1 tablespoon of water. This will give you the added moisture content dry skin needs. Pour into a labeled jar. Shake vigorously before using. For other dry skin advice see Sections 3, 4 and 8.

Herbal Cleansing Waters

Many herbs, either in infusion or in distilled form, help clean the face. They also have healing and soothing powers. You can make these infusions and use them strained, but they do not last long unless you keep them in the refrigerator. For this reason it is useful to be able to buy distilled herbal waters; the British Society of Herbalists have an excellent distilled elder flower water in Caswell-Massey in New York and the Culpeper shops in London.

Elder flower water was once considered an absolute necessity for the complexion, and earlier generations relied on it to keep the skin fair and free of blemishes. It has not lost its reputation among present-day herbalists. The French call it *eau de sureau* and consider it stimulating, cleansing and mildly astringent. Old herbals sometimes call it *aqua sambuci*.

I learned the following recipe from my grandmother, who told me it went back many generations in our family:

buttermilk	½ pint
elder blossoms	5 tablespoons
honey	2 tablespoons

Gently heat the buttermilk and soak the elder blossoms in it. Keep warm and simmering for ½ hour until the blossoms soften. Remove from heat. Steep for 3 hours. Reheat. Strain. Add honey. Keep refrigerated. Use as a face cleanser.

Elder blossoms can also be used in your bath water to soften your skin (see Chapter III).

A recipe for *virgin milk*, with variations and under different names, often appears in old herbals and books of cosmetic lore. Why was it called virgin (sometimes virginal) milk? Possibly because a glass of water becomes pure milky white instantaneously when the tincture of benzoin is added; or because it has such a clearing effect on the skin. Used as a cleanser it will soften and soothe the skin, and it is also an old English remedy for pimples and red spots:

| simple* tincture of benzoin | 15 drops |
| glass of water (spring or distilled if possible) | |

optional

| glycerine | 3 drops |
| tincture of myrrh | 3 drops |

Instead of water you can use rose, orange or elder flower water. In Chapter X you will find an inexpensive recipe for homemade rose and orange water.

A strong infusion of dried pimpernel flowers, *pimpernel water,* may be kept in the refrigerator and used daily as an astringent complexion cleanser. This was another well-known standby, and references to it even appear in Restoration comedy: "Oh, why

---

*Use only simple tincture, not compound tincture. The compound has elements added which are harmful to the skin. If your pharmacist doesn't stock it, ask him to order some, or make some up for you.

does she have such a huge freckle on her face? She should use my pimpernel water!''

Plantain water is another herbal cleanser. Plantain is one of the commonest garden weeds and can be found on most lawns. The Greeks considered it a healing herb. In the Highlands they call it by the Gaelic word *slanlus*, which means "plant of healing." The crushed leaves can be applied directly to the skin for such problems as bites, stings, swellings and bruises. Several ancient herbalist sources mention plantain in combination with other cosmetic healing items such as houseleek and lemon juice, or, as Mrs. Hagger recorded, under "Severall Select Experiments," plantain water mixed with pounded almonds. To make plantain water, add boiling water to the fresh washed leaves and steep for ½ hour or longer. Strain. Refrigerate.

Food Cleansers

A *sunflower seed cleanser,* rich in natural vitamin E and lecithin, is simple to make in small or large quantities. Grind, or blend, 2 tablespoons of sunflower seed kernels to 1 teaspoon of water (preferably distilled or pure mineral water). If you like to experiment, add a scant ¼ teaspoon of honey and ¼ teaspoon of sunflower oil. This will give you a smoother effect, but will be slightly sticky because of the honey.

Normal and oily skin food cleansers. For cleansing normal or oily skin, peeled, grated potato is particularly good. It has been used for centuries to cleanse the skin of impurities and blemishes. It has been claimed to cure eczema. Potato water wash is made by extracting the juice in a vegetable juicer. Make it fresh each day, or keep a large amount in a labeled jar in your refrigerator. Potatoes are healing, cleansing and nourishing for the skin.

Yogurt plus a few grains of salt can also be used by those with oily and normal skin (see Section 6).

Dry skin must be cleansed in a special way. Do not use ordinary soaps, as, although they will remove grime, they contribute to the dry condition. Almond oil and avocado oil are excellent cleansers for those with dry skin. Earlier in this section is a special cocoa butter dry skin liquid cleanser. Natural soaps, glycerine soaps, vegetable soaps and super fatted oatmeal soaps are suitable cleansers. For additional facts on dry skin see Section 8.

Oatmeal, almond meal, cornmeal and bran are still in every day use in many parts of the world as a substitute for soap. In parts of India, a form of cornmeal is used for complexion scrub material and as a cleansing powder, and is brushed through the hair. These meals are all valuable assets in complexion care, since they contain vegetable hormones which nourish the skin.

Any of these meals can be put into a small lidded jar and kept in the bathroom. They are effective with water added to them. For a stronger body scrub, they can be used with a rough wash cloth or loofah. In my home we prefer colloidal oatmeal,* a suspended-particle version of oatmeal, which dissolves easily and leaves the skin with a creamy, silky texture. Those with allergic or adolescent skin will find it efficacious as a body, face and hand "soap."

Lemon is such an obvious cleanser that most people have forgotten about it. But it is truly particularly effective on the hands, and will overcome any strong food odors such as fish or garlic. Since it gets moldy, keep only small amounts in the kitchen or bathroom.

While I was traveling in the west of England, an enchanting lady told me her family lemon-cleansing complexion recipe:

> whole lemon
> rock candy†   several pieces
> gold leaf
> hot ashes

Make a hole in a lemon. Fill the inside with rock candy, and close the cavity with gold leaf. Roast the lemon in the hot ashes of a fireplace, or use charcoal bricquettes in a hibachi barbecue. When you need lemon juice, squeeze out a little through a hole in the gold leaf onto a cloth and wash your face.

She had an exceptionally good complexion and she claimed that the juice not only cleansed her face but brightened it.

---

*Obtain in drugstore.

†Rock candy, pieces of sugar on a string, is used for coughs and is available from old-fashioned drugstores, or by mail order.

Soap

Of all the commercial soaps I prefer those which include glycerine. *Pears* is such a soap. This pure product, which can still be bought in drugstores, goes back many years. A nineteenth-century toiletry book by Anna Kingsford quotes a leading dermatologist of the time as follows: "The more nearly negative a soap is, the nearer does it approach perfection. It is essentially in this respect that *Pears* soap excels. I have reason to think that *Pears* soap is the best because it is the purest ever made, an opinion vouched for by the strictness of chemical analysis. So effectually for medical purposes has the process of purification been carried out, that this soap, when made up in a lather, can be applied to the surface abraded by eczema."

By a "negative" soap she means a soap with as little alkaline content as possible—though it has to have some, or it would not be soap. Fairly neutral negative soaps are made from oatmeal and vegetables, and plants such as aloes and amole. These can be bought at some drugstores or health stores.

Since most home soaps are made with lye, no such recipes are included in this book. If you know of a recipe without lye, and would like to share it, please contact me through the publisher.

Hundreds of growing things contain saponin, a natural soaping ingredient, found in various leaves, flowers, twigs, bulbs, berries and trees.

The best known, and my favorite, soap source is one called by many names, including soapwort. "Wort" is the old English word for plant or herb, and is often found as the final syllable in country names for herbs, particularly those with a medicinal or superstitious application. Soapwort is also known as bouncing Bet, and while it was once a cultivated garden plant only, it now grows wild and can be found in profusion in wastelands. In the American South it is sometimes called my lady's washbowl. It was known to European peasants, and was often used by medieval monks, who called it fuller's herb.

Bouncing Bet or soapwort is a perennial which blooms along roadsides and meadows from July to September. It is a very pretty plant about 2 feet tall with 1-inch pink (sometimes white) flowers which grow in loose clusters. Although the stems contain a gummy juice which will produce a lather, it is the root which is mucilaginous and soapy when agitated in water.

Yucca, Chlorogalum, Lamb's Quarters

These three soapy plants are American Indian discoveries. All are excellent for skin care, or hair shampooing and clothes washing.

Yucca or Spanish bayonet is a striking cultivated plant with spiky, rigid leaves. It also grows wild in the southwest United States, particularly in New Mexico and Arizona. It is called amole in parts of Mexico and there are several amole soaps on the market. Soap made from yucca softens and is most agreeable to the skin. It is useful for clothes washing as well as hair shampoos too.

The rootstock of yucca is rather deep, so you might need a crowbar to uproot it. Use this soap root by breaking into little pieces and washing free of dirt and grit. It can be activated directly in water or in a muslin bag.

Chlorogalum (*pomeridianum*) is a part of the lily family and grows wild in the hilly sections of California. To discover this bulb, look in the late spring for a cluster of stemless, grass-like leaves that later form into a tall spray of widely spread, white, small, lily-like blossoms. These emerge a few at a time in the evening and wither by the next day.

The bulb when dug out looks like a coconut-husk light bulb. Strip the hairy, fibrous coat to find the moist heart 1 or 2 inches wide and 2 to 4 inches long. Crush this *inner* bulb and rub it briskly in water for a wonderful non-alkali shampoo that eliminates dandruff and leaves the hair soft and glossy. This soap dries easily and can be put aside for use months later.

Lamb's quarters or pigweed is a weedy-looking plant with greenish flowers and triangular leaves which turn yellow. The fresh root is deep, spindle-shaped and quite brittle. It is easily crushed into soap form when agitated in water.

Pacific coast *lilac, myrtle, buckbush* are another source of excellent soap. These fresh blossoms provide the rarest of treats—a sort of Polynesian island fantasy good for cleansing and for skin softening.

Be careful when picking these flowers not to pick also the green stalks or you will have a green lather with a funny smell. The green seed vessels can also be used as a soap, but if not rinsed right off leave a yellow stain.

There are three species of tree that have small white flowers and fleshy berries about the size of cherries, which in turn contain one or two seeds that lather in water. I offer the Latin names so that they can be looked up in a tree book. *Sapindus saponaria* can be found on the tip of Florida; *S. marginatus* is an evergreen found along the Atlantic seaboard from the Carolinas to Florida; *S. drummandi* is to be found from Kansas to Louisiana and westward to Arizona. This tree is also called soapberry or wild China tree, as it resembles the true China tree, or jaboncillo (little soap). This tree has clusters of yellow berries, which turn black as they dry and can readily be seen in the bare winter winds until spring.

Those of you who beachcomb should look for the small yellowish split-pea size *eggs* of the *sea snail,* as they are excellent washballs. A sailor friend tells me that many old fishermen and sailors prefer these eggs to ordinary store-bought soap.

3. WRINKLES

Some crinkles and creases are admirable. Don't trade in your smile and eye lines—they establish who you are and how much you laugh and smile! Disregarding genetics, here are six factors which influence the look and texture of your skin. These are all things *you* are in charge of in your life: stress, food, sleep, smoking, drinking and exposure to the sun.

Think of your skin as the ultimate reflector. Whatever you are doing, how you feel, what you eat, how much you sleep, what tensions you are under—all eventually show in the color, texture, vitality and youthfulness of your skin. Food—the fuel your body lives on—has a profound effect on the healthy look of the skin. Sleep is also a controllable factor. If you are sleep deprived, or live with a sleep deficit, it shows under the eyes, and in the tone of the skin.

There are three negative influences on skin that can easily be regulated: *sun* exposure, *smoking* and *alcohol* guzzling. The sun dehydrates and coarsens the skin, and eventually, with too much exposure, produces a map of wrinkles. Also too much sun exposure and sunburn have a *direct effect* on basal cell and squamous cell carcinoma, and are strongly involved in the ultimate skin insult: melanoma, an often-fatal skin cancer. Alcohol and smoking each have a dire effect on one's health and the appearance of the skin. Each puff of nicotine, each drink of alcohol acts in the same

SUNLIGHT AND SKIN CANCER

	CANCERS	RISKS	PREVENTION
ADULTS	BASAL CELL and SQUAMOUS CELL carcinomas appear on sun-exposed skin. CANCER NOT DEADLY—surgery effective and simple	Cancers occur in direct proportion to amount of time spent in sun. There is a cumulative effect—may cause mutation in one gene	Check moles Avoid sunburn Use sunblock, preventive clothing—hat, glasses Stay shade/peak sunlight hours (midmorning to early afternoon)
	MELANOMA can be fatal Increasing in USA— cancer cases double every 10 to 12 years	Be on alert if there is a family link (5–10% have close family connection) 100 or more moles is risk Sunburn may either trigger cancer growth after inflammation or suppress immune system Old exposures to sunburn increases risk	Sunblock, but do not prolong exposure, as there are indirect, and still unknown connections between this cancer and sunlight Wear protective clothing in sun—hat, glasses Keep out of sun during peak hours Use immune aid vitamins/herbs
CHILDREN		Childhood sunburn increases risk of melanoma	Use protective clothing, blocks—**PREVENT SUNBURN!**

way as a bank withdrawal, destroying many milligrams of B and C vitamins, and this breaks down the DNA. This results in coarser, older-looking, crumpled skin.

Other wrinkle provokers are lack of protein, causing a loss of elasticity and tone, which shows up as sagging skin. Further, lack of external (topical) and internal moisture and oils also has a significant impact on wrinkling. To maintain a young-looking skin one must drink a lot of pure water, and ingest some form of unsaturated fatty acid *oil*. Other wrinkle adders are personal "markers"—gestures and grimaces, lifting of eyebrows, furrowing of forehead, frowns and scowls. These create imbedded lines on the face.

Massage Techniques for Applying Creams

Massage the neck and under the chin with upward, outward motions.

Massage the chin area with upward motions, forward and over the jawline towards the ears.

Massage laugh lines upwards, over the upper cheek towards the outer section of the eye.

Delicately pat the under-eye area from nose bridge out to temples.

Gently massage crow's-feet upwards towards the temples.

Massage the forehead from the middle. Stroke upwards with two hands each going in upward, outward motions towards opposite upper temples.

Wrinkle-Chaser Food—Internal

Your skin reflects your general health. By its color and tone, by its bounce, it shows the effect of a diversified diet high in vegetable power, and vegetable juices (especially carrot juice which contains the skin food vitamin A). A run of sleepless nights, pain, and persistent constipation also shows up as reminders on the face.

To resist early wrinkle formation, you must have a varied diet with a complete range of vitamin supplements. You especially need the antioxidants vitamin C, vitamin A, vitamin E and the mineral selenium, all of which quench those small oxygen fires that attack your DNA. Also, nutritional brewer's yeast and kelp will help in keeping the wrinkles at bay. Brewer's yeast comes in four forms: a liquid with oxygen, or as tablets, flakes or powder. This yeast is energizing, is high in all the B vitamin and this in turn helps one to avoid heavy folds and deep wrinkle patterns. Some people initially react to nutritional yeast with a bloated or "gas" effect. This can be adjusted with papaya tablets or hydrochloride tablets with betaine. Cucumber, which has almost the same pH as the skin is thought to also contain a vital antiwrinkle substance. Eat cucumbers in salads, and also apply directly on the skin as an instant facial. It is especially cooling applied cold on closed eyelids.

Lanolin and Vitamin E Moisturizer

Vitamin E, taken internally, increases circulation, so it has a significant secondary effect on the skin. Topically, it is a remarkable healing agent on wounds—even raw wounds, cuts and scars. It is a fine secondary treatment for burn scars (the immediate treatment is ice water). For topical use there are some good vitamin E moisturizers on the market. For instant use for cuts and scars, prick an E capsule and apply. For large areas add a tiny bit of lanolin cream to aid application.

Vitamin Nourishing Cream

My favorite nourishing cream contains both vitamin E and vitamin A, two vital additions to your cosmetic shelf. Use this cream as a skin *food* after you have thoroughly cleansed your skin. Whenever possible use it an hour or two before you go to bed, then wipe it off gently. Whenever you sleep, your skin should be encouraged to breathe free of creams.

beeswax	1½ tablespoons
white wax	1 tablespoon
anhydrous lanolin	1 tablespoon (liquid or solid)
sweet almond oil	3 ounces (avocado oil or safflower oil can also be used)
distilled water	1 ounce
borax	½ teaspoon
rose water	1 ounce (instead of distilled water you can use 2 ounces of rose water)

simple tincture of benzoin (not compound)
2 to 6 capsules of vitamin E (400 I.U.)
2 to 6 capsules of vitamin A (25,000 I.U.)

In a double boiler, heat together the beeswax, the white wax and the lanolin. Slowly add almond, avocado or safflower oil. In a separate pan (glass or stainless steel) heat 1 ounce of distilled water, and the borax (this acts as a special emulsifier) until the borax dissolves completely. Slowly add the rose water so that it too is slightly warm. Now, without allowing either pan to get cool, add the rose water and borax combination to the wax, lanolin and oil combination and beat with an electric beater for as long as it takes for the cream to cool to room temperature. Add the simple tincture of benzoin. Prick open your vitamin capsules, add to cream and beat until the vitamins are blended.

For a nourishing eye cream see Chapter V.

Lily Root and Lanolin Cream Nourisher

Lily and narcissus roots have formidable reputations in complexion and wrinkle care. Use them pulverized with other complexion herbs, honey and rose water to make a complexion water. Make sure they are pesticide free.

water	1 cup
powdered lily roots	2 tablespoons
honey	1 tablespoon
anhydrous lanolin	1 ounce
rose water	½ teaspoon

Add a cup of water to powdered lily root. Simmer in covered pot for ½ hour. Strain and add honey. To make into cream, add an ounce of liquid or solid lanolin melted in a double boiler. Add rose water. Put into a labeled jar.

Avocado Cream Skin Nourisher

whole eggs	2
glycerine	1 teaspoon
lemon juice	½ teaspoon
avocado oil	enough to thicken mixture
sea salt	pinch
cider vinegar	⅛ teaspoon
egg yolks	3
water (or orange or rose)	2 tablespoons

optional

| vitamin A | 50,000 I.U. |
| vitamin E | 400 I.U. |

Blend together fresh eggs, glycerine, lemon juice. Slowly add drop by drop enough avocado oil to thicken the mixture. Add sea salt, cider vinegar. When this is thickened to a cream-like consistency, add beaten egg yolks and the water. Completely blend the mixture. Pour into a labeled jar. This must be kept in a refrigerator.

Sweet Cream Line-Eraser

Sweet cream is a nourishing food for the complexion. Always remember to pat it on in the manner described under massage techniques.

Onto a thoroughly clean skin pat a mixture of a whipped egg white and a teaspoon of cream. Allow to dry for 20 minutes and wash off with tepid water.

Myrrh Facial

Athenian ladies used this wrinkle-prevention facial. It was made by burning powdered myrrh, a powerful healing astringent resin, in an iron plate, allowing the fumes to penetrate the skin of the face. This same effect can be duplicated easily by adding a few drops of tincture of myrrh to any steam facial. Use only on an occasional basis. Myrrh tincture is available in drugstores, and as a resin from botanical sources.

Onion Water

Fresh onions are reputedly marvelous for the skin and can prevent blemishes. Mash, blend or pulverize the onion and use the juice. According to ancient herbalists, the juice can also be added to honey and white wax and used as an antiwrinkle preparation.

Eau de Circe

Circe was the sorceress described by Homer, who turned the companions of Odysseus into swine. Over the years her name has come to be applied to any fascinating or irresistible woman.

In an ancient French toiletry book I found the following recipe for "Eau de Circe." The French considered it an aid in preventing wrinkles. The gum benzoin and the alcohol will tighten and dry the skin, so *don't* use the preparation if you have *dry* skin.

ethyl alcohol (70%)	8 ounces
simple tincture of benzoin	4 drops
melted gum arabic	4 drops
oil of sweet almonds	1 drop
pulverized ground cloves	pinch
ground nutmeg	pinch
rose water	1½ ounces

Pour the alcohol into a clean quart bottle. Add the benzoin, gum arabic, oil of sweet almonds and the cloves and nutmeg. Shake together. Let the preparation stand for a few days, shaking it occasionally; then add rose water. Use it at night before retiring.

4. FACIALS

The aim of a facial mask is to clean, restore, nourish and awaken the skin. The outcome should be a downy, smoother, fresher face. Dozens of simple home products can be used in facials, including healing and skin-restoring household items like honey, milk, yogurt, buttermilk, whey, egg white, egg yolk, lemon, vinegar, hormone-rich cereal and nut meals, vegetable, animal and nut oils, fruits and vegetables, as well as herbal and clay products.

You can experiment by mixing together any of the substances mentioned in this section—unless you have oily or dry skin, in which case note carefully which of the ingredients mentioned are good for your type of skin, and check in Sections 6 and 8, where you will find facials for your specific problem. If your mixture comes out too runny, use any of the following binding substances: banana, honey, fuller's earth, kaolin, almond meal, oatmeal, whole egg; egg yolk for dry skin, egg white, yogurt or buttermilk for oily skin.

Ingredients for Facials

Two easily obtained neutral facial *clays* are kaolin and fuller's earth. Add to any mask to give it more body and firmness. Fuller's earth is an absorbent clay which was originally used by fullers, in cloth mills, to remove grease from fabrics, when the cloth was being cleaned and thickened for the market. (It is also mentioned elsewhere in this book as a dusting powder for feet, and as a dry shampoo for the hair.) Kaolin is the fine white clay used in the manufacture of porcelain.

Yet another useful inert clay for masks is bentonite. Because it is healing and soothing, it is sometimes used by dermatologists for treatment of wounds, sores and eczema.

The *milk and egg products* suggested for facials each have particular uses. Please note the restrictions on all these products; they depend on the quality and texture of your skin. People with normal and youthful skin can use *any* milk or lactic acid milk product, or egg white, egg yolk or whole egg in their facial masks. People with dry skin should only use the lecithin-rich* egg yolk in masks, since egg white is too drying. Dry-skinned people must also restrict their milk soothers, healers and binders to sour cream, sweet cream, skim milk and whole milk. Those with oily skin will learn to appreciate the drying, tightening qualities of beaten egg white, whey and the lactic acid products, buttermilk and yogurt.

Of the many *oils* which can be used as facial nourishers, wheat germ oil, avocado oil and almond oil are preferred. However, you can substitute wheat germ flour, crushed whole avocado, powder from pulverized almonds or the grocery shop emollients, safflower, peanut, canola, corn or olive oil.

The fatty acid GLA (gamma-linolenic acid) enhances healthy skin, hair and nails. It is available for internal use as capsules of unsaturated fatty acids, flaxseed oil, black currant oil, borage oil or evening primrose oil. Internal use of GLA oils adds a youthful glow to the skin, subdues eczema and overcomes brittle hair, fragile nails, dry skin. This same oil helps to control most premenstrual problems. The oil is also a positive factor in arthritis and autoimmune diseases.

Gum resins such as benzoin, tragacanth and arabic are most useful as tightening agents. Benzoin is also a skin cleanser, and can be used in dozens of different facials and creams. Benzoin is soluble in alcohol. To learn how to make an alcohol tincture, see Chapter I. Gum tragacanth is soluble by leaving in water for 24 hours—the ribbon variety dissolves more easily; gum arabic, which comes from Africa, can be dissolved in double its weight of water.

Vegetables and fruits contain a myriad of trace minerals, many enzymes and vitamins. Some have an acid effect on the skin, some are neutral and others are alkaline.

Skin's Acid Mantle

The skin has a certain amount of acidity, called an acid mantle. The pH value is a way of expressing acidity and alkalinity on a

*Lecithin, an invaluable skin aid, can also be obtained in liquid form.

scale from 0 to 14; the skin has a value between 4 and 6, generally taken as 5.5. The acid mantle acts as a protective barrier against infection. A healthy skin produces its own acid mantle within a few hours of washing, but constant washing or swimming can be destructive, and you can help replace the acidity with judicious use of various food products patted on the skin. This is why cider vinegar is such a useful skin aid. Cider vinegar can be drying used undiluted, but used diluted, as it would be in a bath, it is good for any texture of skin and helps normalize it.

The most neutral of the fruits and vegetables are the cucumber, watermelon, fig, raw horseradish, onion, persimmon, sweet green pepper and banana. Tomato is not very acid. The least acid foods, which will be a great help to people with dry skin, are cantaloupe, avocado, honeydew melon, olive, lettuce, carrot. If you need an acid boost to the skin, these are the most acid foods you can use in a facial, starting with the highest acidity: lime, lemon, grapes, cranberry, strawberry, pineapple, grapefruit, apple.

You can use any of the above foods squeezed or patted on the face as you're preparing them to eat. Allow them to dry on the face and wash off with tepid water. If you want a more formal facial, mash up 2 tablespoons of any of the above foods and mix with a binder: honey is a neutral binder; buttermilk, yogurt, clays, earth, egg white are drying binders good for oily skin; banana, sour cream and egg yolks are good binders for dry skin. Always add 5 or 6 drops of cider vinegar; or try adding a dollop of your favorite oil and 2 or 3 drops of cider vinegar to a dry-skin facial.

Other ingredients. Anhydrous lanolin is a good ingredient for attributes, as it attracts water to the skin. Glycerine has the same qualities. Honey is another water-attracting product and is also healing and nourishing for the skin. Buy uncooked honey whenever possible, and use it for creams, facials and special baths.

Cider vinegar can be added to almost any mask. Brewer's yeast can be used in a facial (see Sections 6 and 8 for other uses).

Herbs for Facials

Many herbs are useful for facials. Fennel, nettle, oat flowers, hay flower and lime flowers (linden) can help release impurities from the skin. Use them in the prefacial steaming. Other skin-cleansing herbs are the mild and apple-fragrant chamomile, and lady's mantle. Nettle and rosemary will increase the circulation. Elder flower, horsetail and peppermint are stimulating and tightening for the skin. The best herbs for oily skin are lady's mantle and the very astringent yarrow. When the skin is damaged from too much sun or an infection or wound, use healing herbs such as fennel, houseleek, marshmallow or comfrey. Comfrey has always been known as a wound healer. It contains allantoin, which stimulates cell growth. Its Latin name, *symphytum officinale,* comes from the Greek root meaning "to knit together." Recent research indicates that it is no longer advisable to use comfrey *internally.* However, it can be productively applied in healing facials, and as an ointment to encourage healing of bruises, cuts and scars.

Other gelatinous plants such as Irish moss, quince seed and flaxseed will also soften the skin. These herbs are especially useful additions to clay facial masks, as they help the masks come off more easily. To use, soften small amounts of the herb in hot water, cool, and add to facial.

How to Use Herbs in Facials

All the herbs mentioned may be used in infusion unless otherwise noted. Pour 1 to 2 cups of boiling water over 2 tablespoons, steep for 15 minutes to 3 hours and strain. Use only *1* tablespoon of the herb infusion in the facial; keep the rest for a face wash, or for other uses. Put it in a labeled jar in the refrigerator.

Comfrey contains a great deal of mucilage, which is softening and healing. You can use comfrey by infusing the leaves and adding it to a steam facial; by mashing the fresh leaves and using it as a compress on the face, or by boiling ½ ounce of the crushed root in 1 *quart* of milk or water. Strain and add a tablespoon of either the infusion or the decoction to any facial. External use of comfrey is effective for wounds and sores that are hard to heal.

An infusion can be made from dried fennel fruit; or a decoction from the seed. Use dried houseleek leaves in infusion, or pound fresh houseleek in a marble mortar and squeeze out the juice; pour a few drops of ethyl alcohol or vodka on the juice when you want to use it. It will turn milky.

How to Use a Facial Mask

First cleanse the skin. For a thoroughly deep pore-cleansing before a facial, first steam your face as described in Section 2. If you steam your face, or are going to use a clay or earth mask, or an almond meal or oatmeal mask, which absorb dirt from the pores, you do *not* have to cleanse the skin with a complexion water or cream.

Gently pat the mixed ingredients on to your face. Allow between 15 and 30 minutes for the mask to "take." You can intensify the effect of a mask by lying down quietly with herb-soaked pads covering the eyes, and with your feet higher than your head. Afterwards wash off the mask with cotton pads or a soft washcloth and tepid water. Make sure that the hairline and ears are clean. The pores will be wide open, so close them with a gentle astringent (see Section 13).

Often you will have more than you need for one facial. Some ingredients can be stored in the refrigerator for the next day, but eggs coagulate and many other items harden when mixed together, so you are better off using leftovers immediately as a hand or body rub. Some facial masks make excellent healing and restoring body lotions. They are particularly effective on areas which sometimes have dry or dead skin: the buttocks, the elbows and the backs of the legs.

Honey Circulation Facials

Honey is a remarkably versatile natural product. It acts as a *moisturizing* agent and is therefore particularly good for dry skin. It is also *stimulating, soothing* and *healing.* It can be applied to roughened skin blemishes—alone or in combination with many other natural substances. If you wish, you can add a tablespoon to any facial listed in this book.

The following ingredients mix especially well with honey:

Pulverized almonds, almond oil, almonds and milk.

Avocado, wheat germ, safflower, sesame, peanut, and corn oils.

For normal or oily skin: beaten egg white, or egg white and ¼ teaspoon of either lemon or cider vinegar.

For dry skin: egg yolks, a few drops of cider vinegar, any of the oils mentioned above.

Any complexion herb.

Moisturizing Facials

Every skin can benefit from a moisturizing boost, particularly since sunshine, polluted air and dry centrally heated indoor air removes much of the moisture from the skin.

One of the best moisturizers is vitamin E. Prick a capsule of 100 I.U. (International Units) of this vitamin and smear it on your face often. Since it is rather thick, try to mix it with a little liquefied anhydrous lanolin.

Glycerine is a moisturizer which will extract water from lower tissues of the skin and from the air. You can use glycerine with rose water.

Honey and peach juice are also moisturizers.

Use any of these products in conjunction with such penetrating oils as avocado, wheat germ or almond. Or use safflower, olive or corn oil in your facials.

In making a mask with these materials add any or all of the following ingredients: egg white or egg yolk, or milk products such as sour cream, yogurt, buttermilk, milk, sweet cream, clay products.

Moisturizer-Lotion Mask

This combination of oils and vitamins will sink into your skin and leave it feeling refreshed, soft and moist. It will feed the skin and by helping to keep it elastic prevent the onset of wrinkles. You can occasionally leave the mask on overnight, but not often, as your facial pores should breathe freely while you sleep.

The mask relies on several healing oils and two skin-nourishing vitamins—A and E. Since these are all stable oils you can double or triple the recipe. Use a dark bottle if you can, and be sure to label the contents.

Figures in parentheses are maximum quantities.

wheat germ oil*	1 tablespoon
avocado oil	2 tablespoons
almond oil	1 tablespoon
sesame oil†	2 tablespoons
vitamin A‡	2 capsules (50,000 I.U.)
vitamin E	2 capsules (400 I.U.)

Mix oils together. Prick open capsules and add to oils. Shake vigorously. Label jar. To make a harder mask add clay, honey, egg or a milk product.

Deep Pore Cleansing Clay Mask

beeswax	⅛ ounce
lanolin (anhydrous)	1 ounce
rose water	⅛ pint
fuller's earth	4 ounces

optional

teaspoon of melted quince seed, flax seed (linseed), or Irish moss (carragheen), or teaspoon of unflavored dissolved gelatine: vegetable coloring

This is a famous salon facial mask, one which they charge a lot of money for. The lanolin is a marvellous emollient. The fuller's earth will absorb dirt.

Melt the wax, together with the lanolin, in a double boiler. Add the

*Keep refrigerated to avoid rancidity.
†Do not buy the dark Japanese sesame oil as it smells too strong.
‡Vitamin A is usually made from a fish oil. For a non-fishy odor use one made from palm oil or lemon grass.

rose water and stir thoroughly. Add the vegetable coloring if you want to tint the mask. If you like a scented mask this is the time to add a few drops of your favorite essence or cologne. Stir in the fuller's earth and work all in a mortar until a smooth mixture is obtained.

You can double or triple the quantities in this recipe to make a long-lasting larger batch.

The Spring Peeler Facial

This is a once-in-a-while facial for after the winter, or after an illness or high fever when your face looks sallow and saggy.

Rub your favorite vegetable or nut oil (such as wheat germ oil, avocado oil, almond oil) over your entire face and neck. Immediately pat on gently a drop of warm water and over that pat on a third layer of pure lemon juice. Wait for about a minute, but not long enough for the oil or lemon to dry.

With your index and middle finger start rubbing this emulsion with a circular motion until a little ball forms. Discard the ball and collect another ball until your face looks fresh and peeled.

Papaya Peeler

A steam infusion of papaya tea, or application of papaya juice, will remove dead skin cells from the face. Papaya contains an enzyme which can soften protein tissue. Do not rub it into the skin, as the action of this fruit is quite strong. After steaming, gently wash the face with tepid water and close pores with a mild astringent. If you are using papaya juice straight on the face, wash off after 5 minutes, dry face with a soft cloth, and close pores with a mild astringent.

Pre-Party Facials and Masks

Women have been using mud and food on their faces for thousands of years, and I delight in this quotation from the Roman poet Juvenal, who complains that the Roman husband hardly ever recognizes his wife while she is at home because of her masks, and it is only when she sallies forth to the market, festival or party that:

The eclipse then vanishes, and all her face
Is open'd and restored to every grace
The crust removed, her cheeks as smooth as silk
Are polish'd with a wash of asses milk.

What you want before a party is something to nourish the skin and increase the circulation of your face so that you look particularly bright and glowing. There are many products which can brighten, tingle and enliven the skin temporarily.

Egg-white tightener. Beat 1 egg white and pat on face. It will tighten immediately. Allow to dry for 15 minutes and rinse off with tepid water and cotton wool.

Cinderella make-up tightener. This is a makeup secret told me by a film makeup man. Technically it is not a facial mask but rather a partial facial left on under makeup. It is an under-eye tightener, and is useful for a special party, a photography session or a day when you don't feel at your best and want to look extra special. But alas, as with Cinderella you must leave "the ball" after a few hours, for the tightener only lasts that long.

Beat ¼ of an egg white until frothy. With a thin brush (Japanese writing brushes from artists' suppliers are perfect) paint a very, very thin paste of the egg white under the eyes. The area will tighten. Pat a liquid makeup over the egg white.

Tincture of benzoin circulation booster. This is a cleansing, softening and tightening mask which will make your face tingle and feel more alive.

simple tincture of benzoin	½ teaspoon
glycerine	½ teaspoon
rose water	½ teaspoon
fuller's earth or kaolin	2 ounces

Make a paste of all ingredients. Pat on face with fingers or cotton. Allow the mask to harden for 15 to 30 minutes. Wash off with warm water. Close pores with a mild astringent.

Cereal healing masks. Various cereals have a whitening, softening, soothing effect on the skin. Apply to face or any rough spots on your body.

Use 1 tablespoon of almond paste, almond oil, oatmeal paste or colloidal oatmeal. Blend in a teaspoon of milk, apple pulp, honey or egg yolk. Apply to the face with a patting motion.

Mask for puffy face. There are many anti-inflammatory herbs. Witch hazel extract, chamomile or lady's mantle infusion can be used in a compress, or these same herbs can be added to stiffly beaten egg whites and patted on the face. A stiffly beaten egg white alone can be used to reduce puffiness. A 5-minute mask should be sufficient.

In addition the fatty acid called GLA (gamma-linolenic acid) used internally, acts in an anti-inflammatory manner without any of the side effects of anti-inflammatory drugs. Take *internally* as capsules of either flaxseed oil, black currant oil, evening primrose oil or borage oil.

Russian mask. A modernized version of a mask favored by Russian ladies consists of a tablespoon of healing wheat germ oil, a whipped egg yolk, and a few drops of cider vinegar. Pat on face. Allow to dry for 15 minutes. Wash off with tepid water.

Allergic Skin Facial

wheat germ oil (or flour)	1 tablespoon
yogurt	1 tablespoon

Mix the oil (or flour) and yogurt together until smooth. Pat on face and neck. Allow to dry for 15 minutes. Remove gently with a large, smooth towel or with cotton wool dipped in tepid water. Close pores with an astringent such as rose water or cucumber. Never rub sensitive skin.

Antiwrinkle Facials

No amount of herb facials will be effective for wrinkles without the right diet (see Section 3). But herbs can soften and lubricate the skin, and help in cell regeneration.

Four herbs in particular—comfrey, fennel, houseleek and marshmallow—have been used for centuries both as healing herbs and in the fight against the encroachment of time. See *How to Use Herbs in Facials* (page 30) for ways of using comfrey, fennel and houseleek.

Houseleek is a fibrous root herb which grows on the walls of houses and even on the roofs. In the past it was used as an instant first aid. The juices from the leaves were used to cure scalds and heal sores. It was the favorite herb of Ninon de Lenclos, the renowned French beauty and wit who was born in 1620 and died in 1705, still beautiful. Her nightly facial consisted of the expressed juice of fresh houseleek added to lanolin and almond oil. It is also an excellent herb for skin inflammations and a treasured remedy for pimples. The Greek physician Galen recommended houseleek even for erysipelas and shingles. You can add the juice of the houseleek to any nourishing ointment.

Marshmallow is another herb with softening agents. The dried roots, boiled in water, give out half their weight of a gummy substance similar to starch. Or you can soak an ounce of the roots in cold water for half an hour and then peel off the bark, cut up the root, and soak for a few more hours.

The Duchess of Alba Antiwrinkle Facial

The handsome Duchess of Alba left some interesting stories about her life and loves, as well as an eternal record of her beauty in Goya's painting.

According to the diary which contained this recipe, it could be used as both a facial and a night mask. "This will not only keep out the wrinkles and preserve the complexion fair, but it is a great remedy where the skin becomes too loosely attached to the muscles, as it gives firmness to the parts." However, although this is an antiwrinkle mask, the alum and egg whites are tightening and drying, so it is more suitable for *oily* skin than for those with a tendency towards dry skin.

egg whites	2
rose water	to cover
alum powder	pinch
oil of sweet almonds	¼ teaspoon

Beat egg whites and simmer gently in rose water. Gradually add alum powder and almond oil. Beat all these ingredients together until they assume the consistency of a paste.

Vegetable and Fruit Masks

The healthy skin is slightly acid. The scientific way this is expressed is in the symbols pH (potential of hydrogen) which actually means the degrees of acidity or alkalinity. Neutral pH is 7. The skin has a pH of 5.5. Cucumber, which is cooling and is thought to have special antiwrinkle substances, and papaya are the best match for skin pH. Watermelon, persimmon, casaba melon and banana are also useful in facial masks. Honey is neutral, and in addition to being an excellent binder for other mask substances, it softens and heals the skin.

If your skin needs an acid boost because of excess oiliness, these are the most acid foods you can use in a facial: lime, lemon, grape, cranberry, strawberry, pineapple, grapefruit, apple, all in descending order.

Those with dry skin will want less acid foods and they are: cantaloupe, avocado, honeydew melon, olive, lettuce, carrot and parsley. Parsley is also quite effective with oily skin.

You can use any of the foods mentioned as a spontaneous facial, even as you are preparing salads and desserts. Allow the substance to dry on the face just as you would a real facial, and wash it off with tepid water.

For a ''formal'' vegetable or fruit facial, peel and mash any of the above foods and add to a binding substance. For excessively oily skin you might want to concentrate on drying substances such as buttermilk, yogurt, clay, earth, egg white. Add a few *drops* of apple cider vinegar.

For dry skin banana, honey, sour cream or egg yolk are quite helpful. Add a tablespoon of your favorite oil, and a few *drops* of apple cider vinegar.

Hot-Weather Cucumber Mask

ice cube	
peeled cucumber	
honey	½ teaspoon
milk	2 tablespoons
(for additional thickening add ½ teaspoon powdered milk)	
witch hazel extract	½ teaspoon
peppermint extract or	5 drops
peppermint oil	2 drops

Blend and crush ice cube, cucumber, honey, milk, witch hazel and peppermint. Pat mask on face. Dry for 15 minutes or more, wash off with tepid water, pat dry. Close pores with ice-cold astringent. (Unless you have a sensitive skin or broken veins on face, in which case you must use only a mild astringent.) This is a refreshing, cooling summer mask.

Tightening Cucumber Mask

peeled cucumber	
cider vinegar or lemon juice	¼ teaspoon
witch hazel extract	1 teaspoon
ethyl alcohol	1 teaspoon
egg white	1

Extract the juice of cucumber in a juicer or blend 1 small cucumber quickly (otherwise it liquefies too much in the blender) and add either cider vinegar or pure lemon juice, witch hazel extract or ethyl alcohol.

Take the mixture out of the blender and add 1 whipped egg white. Pat this mixture on the face and allow it to dry for 15 minutes or more. Wipe off with tepid water and a soft washcloth. Pat dry. Pat on herbal or favorite astringent.

Two other optional *tightening* products for this or *any* other mask would be ¼ teaspoon of simple tincture of benzoin, or a pinch of alum powder.

Carrot Mask

Carrots are rich in vitamin A, which is very useful in treating all skin problems and allergy attacks. If you have a persistent skin problem you should explore the benefits of eating lots of raw carrots and drinking carrot juice. A fresh carrot-juice cocktail from an extractor-juicer is a quick pick-me-up too. If you are lucky enough to live where you can obtain pesticide-free carrots they will taste different from most carrots in the market. They are much sweeter and there is absolutely no taste of chemicals.

On a daily basis it is useful to drink the juice of two large carrots. Five large carrots a day is equivalent to 25,000 I.U. of beta-carotene (the water-soluble precursor of vitamin A). Unless there is a specific need for additional vitamin A in the diet, this is considered a high dose. To make a carrot-juice or pulp facial, add either whipped egg white or honey or buttermilk.

Parsley Facial

Parsley adds sheen, and cuts down on excess oiliness of the skin. It is too harsh to rub on the skin, but can be simmered in a small amount of water, cooled and strained, and added to facials. It can also be juiced in a juicer machine. Apple and the skin-helper carrot juice are good additions to parsley facials. To thicken thin juices for facial use, slowly add small amounts of buttermilk, sour cream, yogurt, honey, egg white or egg yolk, or the clays, kaolin or fuller's earth. Apportion the amount depending on the dryness or oiliness of your skin.

Eruptions on the skin can be cured by cleansing the system. One excellent remedy is a consistent use of the combined juics of carrot, parsley, and celery.

Ovid's Beautifying Facial

Have you ever wondered how the ladies of antiquity took care of their skin-nourishing problems? Ovid recorded the following ingredients in a recipe, saying: "Every woman who covers her face with this will make it more brilliant than a mirror."

I like this recipe, but Ovid uses such large amounts that an entire girl's school could take a facial at the same time, so I merely list his ingredients.

Ovid advises the following: lentils, eggs—ground into a powder and then a flour and passed through a sieve (try powdered eggs). Add powdered narcissus bulbs (these and other bulbs mentioned through this book are excellent cosmetic aids), gum benzoin (you could use simple tincture of benzoin), honey and wheat flour.

Gardener's Special Facial

This complexion mask was reported to be effective in producing a bright and pure-looking skin. It will undoubtedly appeal to gardeners, for it relies on equal amounts of the seed of melon, pumpkin, gourd and cucumber. The seeds must be dried and then pounded until they are reduced to a powder. Add enough cream to make this flour into a paste and add enough milk to dilute it. For aroma you might want to add a few drops of lemon oil, or some other aromatic oil. Pat on face. Keep the mask on for 15 minutes or more. Wash off with tepid water. Close pores with astringent.

Other special masks for skin problems, including spots, dry skin, large pores, oily skin, broken (thread) veins, rough skin, or double chin, can be found under the appropriate headings, or by consulting the index.

5. SPOTS

Blackheads, Whiteheads, Pimples, Acne

"Out, damned spot!" Most of us have stood in front of a mirror at some time and wished that a "spot" would disappear. No one likes whiteheads, blackheads or pimples, particularly the kind that can lead to acne.

To cure these blemishes you have to know their cause. Your 21 square feet of skin has many important functions. Besides helping you to breathe and exude perspiration (1 quart a day and up to 20 quarts if you are exercising or tense), it also helps to eliminate toxic material through its millions of pores. Which is why you sometimes get pimples when your stomach is upset. Your skin also reflects your feelings—gooseflesh when you are cold or scared, and pimples when you are unhappy or tense. Your complexion is a reflection of the total you—how much good sleep you have, the food you are eating or not eating, your feelings, your ability adequately to discharge waste materials and your cleanliness.

But this doesn't explain the trauma of sudden and disastrous attacks of whiteheads, blackheads and pimples when young people reach puberty. At the time you care most about your clean and healthy looks, nature somehow foils you. How? Your body has a natural oil-manufacturing system which exudes sebum—nature's cold cream. Too much sebum and your skin is oily. Too little sebum and your skin is dry.

During adolescence there is a great stirring of both female and male hormone production, and if there is the *slightest* imbalance of these hormones, the sebaceous glands are forced to send up *extra* sebum. That would be all right if you could just wipe off this excess oil. But it comes up through the pores, and if there is some sebum stuck there already, you get a white "bump" which, if not almost immediately removed by either steam facial, gentle friction or an enriching oatmeal or other exfoliating scrub, hardens in 7 or 8 hours. The hardened oil is called a whitehead and becomes a blackhead when oxidized by the air.

Sometimes the excess sebum emerges only *under* the skin and causes a reddish bump which, if not immediately cleared, becomes infected when the body's defense apparatus, the white corpuscles, create those most dreaded of all adolescent scourges—pus-filled pimples. A few of these and you have acne. And if you touch your face a lot, and don't keep it scrupulously clean, or if the pus oozes out, the acne spreads.

Girls are frequently troubled by such pimples a few days before their menstrual period when the female hormone production of estrogen is low and the male hormone androgen takes over and causes a slight imbalance. Boys are the worst sufferers from this sudden production of sebum, since male puberty brings on an excess production of male hormones.

Certain foods and vitamins can regulate excess secretions of the skin; among them calves' liver is a good choice. But a word of warning. The function of this organ is to detoxify—therefore animal liver will retain pesticides as well as growth hormones from its feed. Wise consumers purchase *organic* (pesticide-free) liver, or organic liver tablets. Nutritional yeast also helps to adjust skin secretions and is available in flake, powder, tablet and liquid form. B complex vitamins are a necessary adjunct to rebalancing the body secretions. Take at least one a day B complex vitamins in 50 or 100 mg tablets, especially if you smoke or drink alcohol, are on a diet, or have an erratic, stressful schedule. Small amounts of chromium in a multivitamin helps in decreasing infections of the skin. Zinc gluconate (30 mg a day) helps to heal and prevent scars. Unsaturated fatty acid capsules help to make the other vitamins work better, and encourage internal healing.

Another really effective acne aid is *lecithin,* which emulsifies and breaks down fatty globules in the blood. This frequently works wonders. One grown man I know was able to control serious acne on his body with doses of lecithin after failing with every other treatment. The suggested daily dose is 2 tablespoons of the granules dissolved in some fruit juice, or 6 capsules. You can combine the lecithin and the yeast and drink them together.

Herbal drinks and *vegetable juices* are also very useful in clearing blemishes. Carrot juice can be drunk alone—up to a pint a day—or combined with spinach; use about twice as much carrot juice as you do spinach. Or you can use a combination of carrots, lettuce and spinach, in the proportions 5 ounces of carrots, 2 of lettuce, ½ ounce of spinach. Or increase the spinach to 1 ounce and add ½ ounce of parsley. A simple but amazingly effective treatment is lots and lots of *water*—8 to 10 glasses a day.

Acne Don'ts

If you are worried about acne, eliminate these foods from your diet: *fatty* or *fried* foods, most *nuts, animal fat* foods, particularly *butter; shellfish* and *iodized salt,* both of which contain iodine, a substance that stimulates acne. Other no's are *chocolate, cocoa,* sticky *puddings, pork* products, *pies* and *pastries* of all kinds, *Coca-Cola* (but you can use small amounts of Classic Coke, or pure Coke syrup (Heritage Products) to cure diarrhea!) and other *soft drinks, sharp cheeses, dates, sugar, homogenized milk. Alcohol and hot coffee* or *hot tea* dilate the capillaries of the face and should not be used.

Other Causes of Acne

Some infections in the system cause acne—so if you are doing all the right things and your acne is still spreading, have your doctor check your tonsils and your dentist check your teeth. Most people find that large amounts of vitamin C help to clear up chronic infections. Timed-release spansules work well.

Worry and tension are known to increase acne outbreaks. Check other parts of the book for suggestions on easy relaxation exercises and simple sleep aids.

Exercise—indoor and outdoor—can dissipate tension. Yoga exercises are being increasingly accepted here in the West as a method of achieving body control, harmony and relaxation. If there are no classes in your area, you can obtain books and records which will help you to learn the various movements, stretches and breathing methods.

Blackhead and Whitehead Cleansers

The best *de*fense is *off*ense. If you are prone to blackheads and/or whiteheads, try some of these night-cleaning, skin-toning remedies. All of them have been known for generations, and some for many centuries, and were used effectively and happily in the simpler past. Some are preventives, some are preventive-cleansers. All work. You have to experiment and see which one of them suits your temperament and your skin.

Herbal Steam Facial

One of the easiest of all blackhead cleansers is one which my mother learned from her mother and which had been passed down for generations. It is the simple and effective herbal facial (steam) bath.

Boil a pint of water and pour over 2 tablespoons of *any* complexion herb. Suggested herbs are chamomile, yarrow, lady's mantle, nettle, fennel, comfrey, houseleek, lime flowers. Improvise a towel tent-hood and allow the steam to penetrate your face for 10 minutes or more. Your pores should then be wide open and the blackheads can be pushed out by circling them with clean cotton wool or tissue. Do not touch the blackheads with your hands. Close pores with cool water or astringent. If the blackheads are still imbedded in your pores, take a long steamy bath (Epsom salt baths are a help) and then try using the herbal steam facial again. The blackheads will probably come out more easily. For more resistant blackheads, try the almond oil facial or the Never-Fail Blackhead Remover below.

Almond Oil Facial

Gently pat sweet almond oil over the area of visible blackheads. Apply hot towels on the blackhead area several times. Used with the bath and the facial, this will soften deeply imbedded blackheads, and will help loosen them enough for you to push them out with a tissue or cotton wool.

Never-Fail Blackhead Remover

An emergency remover when everything else has failed is the following special facial on the visible blackheads (after you have already opened your pores with a steam facial and bath):

Epsom salts	1 tablespoon
iodine (preferably white)	3 drops
boiling water	1 cup
washcloths	several

Dissolve Epsom salts and iodine in the boiling water. Keep the water piping hot by using an electric kettle, thermos or an electric hot tray. Soak a clean cloth or washcloth in the hot Epsom salt solution and then press on imbedded blackhead area. Change cloth for hot one when cloth cools. To remove blackhead or whitehead, press with a tissue or handkerchief on the outer edge of the blemish. It should pop right out. Close each opened pore with cool water and witch hazel splash.

Honey Cleanser

Honey is a splendid blackhead and facial cleanser as well as skin nourisher and healer. Heat about 4 tablespoons of honey and gently pat over blackhead area or entire face. If your face is particularly blemished, add a small amount of wheat germ to the honey, which will draw the blemishes to the surface of the skin. Honey-Wheat Germ Mask is antiseptic and toning. Keep on face 15 minutes or more. Relax while you wait. Wash off with clean cloth and tepid water. Close pores with astringent. Honey can also be used with the following cereal scrubs.

Cereal Scrubs

Blackheads can also be expelled with a nourishing oatmeal or almond-meal paste mask. You can cook up some old-fashioned oatmeal as if you were making porridge, following the directions on the packet, then add almond meal and gently plaster your face with this paste. You can use this as a daily scrub, as did many famous beauties of the past.

A modern version of the oatmeal scrub is colloidal oatmeal. This needs no prior preparation. Just add water and use as your nonallergenic daily scrub. This is marvelous for people with delicate or allergic skin. There are also oatmeal ''soaps'' on the market which contain no soap and are excellent for allergic skin or persistent skin rashes.

Another old-fashioned mixture which uses *three* blackhead cleansers and preventers is a combination of 3 tablespoons of colloidal oatmeal, a teaspoon of white wine and a teaspoon of lemon. This can be used several times a day. Lemon attracts mold, so make it up fresh, or keep the scrub in the refrigerator, in which case you can make up a larger batch.

Yet another blackhead cleanser combines 4 ounces of powdered colloidal oatmeal with 2 ounces of powdered almond meal, ½ ounce of fuller's earth and about an ounce of a liquid herbal soap or glycerine soap shavings. You can keep this in an attractive container in your bathroom and use it as a liquid scrub by adding water. Rub gently into the blackhead area to make a lather.

Lemon Cleansers

You will find lemon juice, by itself or combined with other products, an ideal blackhead preventer, as it is antiseptic and cleansing, and restores acidity to the skin. Use fresh strained lemon juice whenever you can, or mix with equal parts of rose water or orange or elder flower water.

An effective lemon and whipped egg-white preparation was used for centuries for control of blackheads and for complexion care. Juice ½ lemon. Strain. Whip up an egg white. Heat together in a basin or stainless steel pan until they thicken. Place in jar, label, *and keep refrigerated.* To preserve it without refrigeration, simply add 3–4 drops of simple tincture of benzoin.

Milk

Milk is very useful in blackhead prevention. In fact Dr. Anna Kingsford, a knowledgeable doctor of the late 19th century, wrote that "the only way permanently to rid the face of blackheads is to wash with water as warm as possible, and bathe the face (with a sponge) for 10 minutes in *tepid* milk."

A skin-soothing *herbal milk* can be made by soaking 4 table-spoons of yarrow or chamomile in 2 cups of cold milk for several hours. Keep refrigerated and heat slightly before using as wash.

Lanolin Pimple Cleanser Cream

rose water	1 cup
peeled apple	2 chunks
celery	1 tablespoon
fennel	1 teaspoon
barley meal	2 pinches or ½ teaspoon
egg white	1
anhydrous lanolin	¼ teaspoon

Simmer together, in 1 cup of rose water, the apple, celery, fennel, barley meal. Discard the celery. Add beaten egg white and lanolin. Squeeze the mixture through a strainer, beat until smooth. Place in labeled jar in refrigerator.

Camphor Cucumber Pimple Drying Mask

(This can also be used as a circulation-boosting mask.) Camphor USP* contains a soothing and drying ingredient.

camphor USP	¼ cake
egg white	1

*Camphor USP is a natural camphor, obtainable from drugstores—not mothballs, which are made from a synthetic chemical not to be used on the skin.

peeled cucumber	1
lemon juice	¼ teaspoon
witch hazel extract	2 teaspoons
peppermint oil or extract	3 drops

optional

simple tincture of benzoin	5 drops
or	
powdered alum	¼ teaspoon

Crush camphor, add to whipped egg white and cucumber. Blend together. Add lemon juice (or cider vinegar), witch hazel, peppermint oil or extract. Blend again. For extra tightening action add simple tincture of benzoin or powdered alum. Put mask on face. Allow to dry. Remove in 15 or 20 minutes. Wash off with tepid water. Rinse again. Close pores with strong astringent.

Additional Blemish Controllers

Fresh foods: Pat cucumber slices or juice, or crushed watercress leaves or juice on the face each night and wash off by morning.

Herbs: The following herbs can be simmered as a decoction, strained and patted on the face. Let the liquid dry. Wash off after 15 minutes. Decoction: In water simmer either horsetail, oak bark, silverweed, leaves or roots of gladwin. Simmer wormwood in vinegar.

Salve: Rue flowers and myrtle leaves crushed together and added to an ointment or cream.

Powder: Crushed lupin seeds.

Sap: Daisy juice from stalk—in spring. Slit the bark of willow or birch in spring to release sap. In *Delights for Ladies* by Sir Hugh Platt (1600), I found the following under the charming heading, "A Secret Not Known To Many":

To Take Away Spots and Freckles From the Face and Hands
The sappe that issueth of a Birch tree in great abundance, being opened in March or April, with a receiver of glasse set under

the boring thereof to receive the same, doth perform the same most excellently and maketh the skin very cleare.

Infusion: Pimpernel, patience, alone or combined. Red clover.
Compound: Touch each acne pimple with compound spirit of horse-radish.

Blemish Controls

The following will flush the system of impurities, and release stored fluid and stimulate the kidneys: an infusion (or soup) of fresh parsley, or small one-inch or so bits of red watermelon pulp eaten throughout the day, or a helping of lightly steamed asparagus, or 16 drops of asparagus tincture in water, are excellent foods for the release of stored fluid in the body. Other herbs to increase the flow of urine are decoctions of bread of Indian corn, silver mantle, couch grass.

Freckles

There are two kinds of freckles—sun freckles, which come and go, and chronic or "cold" freckles. You can bleach freckles with various foods and herbs.

Bleaches

All herbal and food bleaches tend to be drying for the skin. To make sure your face and hands don't get too dry from these treatments, oil the freckle area afterwards, unless you already have an oily skin.

Pat any of the following "lotions" on the face or hands and allow to dry from 15 minutes to 1 hour. Wash off with tepid water. Pat dry again. Close pores with gentle astringent. Pat on oil or nourishing cream.

Buttermilk is a gentle bleach.
Equal parts of lemon juice mixed with either elder flower or rose water.

Two tablespoons of grated fresh horseradish in cider vinegar and made into a paste.

Two tablespoons of grated fresh horseradish simmered in milk. Make up into a paste.

Fruits and vegetables with high vitamin C content can also be used to bleach freckles. Make a paste mask of rose-hip powder and small additions of the juice of either parsley, potato, lemon, strawberry or cucumber. Pat on face. Allow to dry. Remove with warm water after 15 minutes. Oil face and use nourishing cream afterwards.

Bleaching herbs that can be used in facials or in infused complexion water are: lime flowers, elder flowers, lady's mantle and chickweed. Any lactic acid product added to elder flower distilled water or elder flower infusion will increase the whitening action of the elder flower. Pat on face. Allow to dry. Wash off with tepid water 15 minutes later. Use cream afterwards.

Brown Spots

Brown spots are a normal part of the aging process and are possibly due to the depletion of certain vitamins, and the rapid breakdown of the cells from free radical "fires." One way to control proliferation of the spots is prompt use of the antioxidant vitamins E, and C, and the mineral selenium. Antioxidants quench the oxygen fires as cells break down the DNA and are renewed. B complex, in the amounts of 50 or 100 mg is also needed.

For freckles, Dr. Jarvis in *Folk Medicine* recommends applying castor oil until the spots disappear.

Moles

Moles are raised brown bumps. They are similar to freckles, both being due to uneven pigmentation. It is said that everyone has at least one little mole.

Most moles are harmless. If a new one appears after the age of 40, check it out for jagged edges, mottled color, flat but larger than a pencil eraser size. If a mole enlarges suddenly, especially with an irregular border, darkens or is inflamed, shows spotty color changes, or begins to bleed, ulcerate, itch or be painful, it should be examined by a dermatologist.

6. OILY SKIN

Oily skin may be hard to control, but it does have the virtue of keeping wrinkles away for a long, long time. Oiliness comes from excess sebum when a slight imbalance within the system forces the sebaceous glands to send up more oil than is needed.

There are many ways of controlling an oily skin: from *within* by changing food habits to exclude rich and fried foods, and to include more greens and certain herbs; and from *without* by daily herbal steaming, deep pore scrubbing with herbs and grease-cutting foods which absorb dirt and grease, and with herbal and food astringents which degrease the face and body and close the pores after cleansing. The best internal emulsifier is lecithin, a by-product of soy beans. Take 2 tablespoons of lecithin granules daily.

Since many adolescents have an oily skin and consequently have trouble with blackheads, whiteheads and pimples, as well as acne, I have included a more complete discussion of this problem in Section 5 of this chapter.

Herbal Steam Facial

Steaming is very good for an oily skin, as it cuts the external grease and deep-cleans the clogged pores, and allows you to push out the blackheads and whiteheads easily, and therefore to avoid pimples.

A description of the steam facial can be found in Section 2.

Cleaners

Fuller's earth can be used to absorb excess oil on the face. Better still are any number of absorbent cereals, which can be used as daily scrubs for the face and body. These include bran, oatmeal, almond meal and cornmeal. Colloidal oatmeal (suspended and ready to use as it is) makes a marvellous, non-allergenic scrub which will leave your skin velvety smooth.

Oily Skin Helpers

Oily skin responds to many easily obtained household products, among them lemon juice, diluted apple cider vinegar, and tepid milk (which also is a useful daily cleanser and blackhead preventer). White wine can be splashed on the skin after cleansing. These other foods can also be applied directly to the skin or added to astringent herbs: buttermilk, beaten egg white, yogurt. Astringent herbs to cut excess skin lubrication are the ancient plant horsetail, which makes up into a stimulating *wash* for oily skin, and washes made up of infusions of yarrow, chamomile, lady's mantle, elder flower or sage. Early herbalists set much store by daily drinks of the astringent herb yarrow to cut down on excessive skin oiliness. Prepare 1 tablespoon of yarrow to a cup of boiling water, steep and strain, and drink warm or cold. (Do not take if pregnant.)

Oily Skin Masks

Cucumber, parsley and cabbage are all excellent in controlling oily skin, but cucumber is the easiest to use. Two other foods which are reliable are tomato and buttermilk, both of which can be used in connection with other ingredients in a facial. Yogurt can also be used as a mask-binder and combined with these foods or the herb infusion we have mentioned before. See Sections 4, 7 and 13.

Tomato-Lemon

This is a real winner for oily skins, as it combines two astringent, skin-nourishing foods. Blend them together in a blender, *or* steep the tomato juice or pulp in the inside of a lemon. After steeping, scrape off the lemon-tomato pulp and splash on your face.

If you haven't time for a whole mask and tend to have an oily skin, rub the pulp of a tomato or lemon on your face, and wash off with tepid water.

Brewer's Yeast Facial

This facial is very successful for those with oily skins and can be used as a tingling, vitamin-rich, nourishing stimulator twice a week. Stir the yeast powder or flakes into a stiff paste with milk, buttermilk, yogurt, rose water, witch hazel, fuller's earth or kaolin, and pat onto a clean face. Wash off with tepid water and close the pores with strong cold astringent.

Marie Antoinette's Oily Skin Mask

Old records show that Marie Antoinette was worried about her too-oily skin. She helped keep it under control with this nightly facial:

milk	½ cup
lemon juice	1 teaspoon
brandy	1 teaspoon

Simmer over a gentle flame. Apply to face. Allow to dry. Wash off 15 minutes later with warm water. Rinse with slightly cooler water. Close pores with astringent.

The Duchess of Alba Facial is also good for oily skin; see pages 37–38.

Astringents

There is a complete listing of herb and food astringent substances in Section 13.

7. LARGE PORES

Although large pores are frequently identified with excess sebum, even people with dry skin can have large pore areas on their face. You can keep the problem under control with steam and herbal facials, which will keep the area clean. In addition, a number of foods and herbs can temporarily tighten the pores.

Any one of the following can be used alone or in combination with each other: beaten egg white, buttermilk, tomato, cornmeal, oatmeal, bran, almond meal, lemon, vinegar and water, alum powder, milk, honey, camphor USP, or the herbs horsetail, sage or yarrow. If you find the herbal mash too watery, add a facial pack thickener like fuller's earth. Clean and dry face before applying the mask. Dry mask on the face for 20 minutes. Afterwards wash off with tepid water and soft cloth. Pat dry. Close pores with astringent. Herbal and other astringents will be found in Section 13.

If you have a dry skin, be sure to use these facials and washes only on the large-pore area of your face.

Egg-White Masks

Frothy egg white is one of nature's most successful skin tighteners and drying agents, thus useful for large pore control. Use egg white alone, or in combination with lemon juice or yarrow infusion, or both.

The peppermint extract adds a decided tingle to this simple egg-white and cucumber mask.

peeled cucumber	½
egg white	1
lemon juice	½ teaspoon
ethyl rubbing alcohol (buy best brand)	1 tablespoon
ice cube	
peppermint extract	4 drops

Peel half a cucumber. Whip up the egg white for a few seconds. Blend the cucumber and egg white, lemon juice, alcohol, ice cube and peppermint extract.

Peppermint creates a menthol effect. If you desire an even

tighter effect from the mask, purchase some alum powder (drugstore or botanical sources), and add a pinch to this recipe.

Another splendid skin tightener is gum arabic, available through herb stores and botanical resources. Use 1 teaspoon in 1 ounce of water. The gum absorbs heated water, doubling its weight.

Tomato Mask

Tomatoes have a lot of vitamin C and potassium, and are very successful in controlling large pores. You can try squishing a tomato on your face, or use buttermilk, or yogurt, or fuller's earth added to the pulp to make a facial paste. Apply to clean face, allow to dry for 15 minutes. Wash off with tepid water.

Buttermilk Washes

Use a 15-minute facial and rinse off carefully. Or buttermilk and salt can be blended together to make a paste.

Large Pore Herb Helpers

A wide variety of herbs help to control large pores. Among them, camphor USP heals, soothes, and tightens the skin. This is natural camphor mind you, not mothballs, a synthetic chemical that must not be used near the skin. Purchase camphor ice, or a bottle of spirits of camphor, add a small amount of either substance to rose water or elderflower water. Apply nightly after cleansing the face. A great facial for large pores is made up of 1 tablespoon of honey, 1 tablespoon of brandy, and 3 drops of spirits of camphor. Apply this mask to the face with special care to avoid getting near the eyes.

Yarrow, horsetail and sage are also helpful for large pores either as internal drinks, or as ingredients in facial masks. For a facial, make a strong infusion by adding a cup of boiling water to 2 tablespoons of any of the herbs. Steep for at least 15 minutes. Strain, add honey, lemon, cider vinegar or alum, or other substances mentioned as an aid to large-pore control.

Almond Meal

Pulverized almond meal has a healing, soothing and nourishing effect on the skin. It was used in ancient Greece for facials and hand creams. The meal comes already prepared, or grind a few almonds by hand or in a grinder. To make a paste for a facial mask, add a few drops of rose water or elder flower water and either milk, buttermilk or yogurt. For even stronger astringency or cleansing, add drops of simple tincture of benzoin.

Cornmeal/Oatmeal Mask

Both oatmeal and cornmeal are softening and nourishing deep-pore cleansers. To make a mask create a slightly thick paste of warm oatmeal or cornmeal. For large pores add liquids such as buttermilk, tomato pulp, cucumber juice, egg white or yarrow, sage or horsetail infusion.

Large Pore Astringent

This will help correct coarse large pores, oily or flabby skin:

cucumber juice	1½ ounces
cologne	1 ounce
elder flower water	5 ounces
simple tincture of benzoin	½ ounce

Mix the cucumber juice, cologne and elder flower water and place in an 8-ounce bottle. Add simple tincture of benzoin. Shake slightly.

8. DRY SKIN

People with dry skin do not produce enough sebum, the internal skin oil. This has an up side, since excessive production of sebum is one of the basic causes of acne. Therefore people with dry skin are spared the discomfort and misery of acne pimples. But later on, as the years advance, this plus turns into a minus, for the lack of lubrication from within the body can lead to a parched looking skin which wrinkles easily. But do not despair, there are solid nutritional and topical solutions to the problem. It is never too late to start on a constructive program of oiling and moisturizing your inner body and outer skin. Moisturize from within by drinking a lot of pure water each day, and feed your body and skin by taking one or another form of unsaturated fatty acid oils or GLA, which nourishes skin, hair and nails. Externally, pat on oil-based products—there are several excellent oils produced by Heritage Products in Virginia. To retain additional oil and moisture, after bathing, blot off excess water and apply *oil* while the skin is *damp*. This regimen and a solid routine of appropriate nutrition will give you results in a short while.

Nutritional Aids

A properly structured nutritional program frequently shows results in less than 2 weeks' time. However, it requires patience for a complete restoration of the skin. It won't be enough to cream and moisturize your face. You must eat a wide variety of vitamins A, B complex C and E-rich *foods*. If your skin is exceptionally dry, or if you are over 40 years old, also add these same vitamins to your diet in the form of supplements, remembering that supplements are just what they say they are—not substitutes for good food.

People on fat-free diets often discover that as they lose weight the facial skin begins to sag. Many nutritionists suggest it is a mistake to be on a completely fat-free diet, that it is necessary and advisable to *add* a moderate amount of monounsaturated oils such as olive, or polyunsaturated oils such as safflower, sunflower and sesame, to the diet. These oils help metabolize the fat-soluble vitamins A and E, and water-soluble vitamin B. The Omega 3 oil in particular acts like an invisible but necessary partner to all the B vitamins and gets them to work for you. In fact, your body cannot manufacture the B vitamins in your intestines without some fat.

Dry-Skin Facial Materials

Many foods are moisturizing as well as nourishing and penetrating. For dry skin care, use the following substances alone or in combination with other suggested materials:

The oil of avocado, wheat germ, almond and linseed (flaxseed) and the everyday oils such as the monounsaturated olive oil or the polyunsaturated safflower and peanut oils, are all useful in dry skin care. Other dry skin helpers are lanolin, egg *yolk,* apple juice, peach juice, sour cream, honeydew melon juice, brewer's yeast, milk, honey, oatmeal, almond meal, crushed almonds and liquid lecithin.

Brewer's Yeast Plan

Brewer's yeast can be helpful to people with either dry or oily skin, since it helps control skin secretions. It is a source of all the B vitamins. Since some skin deficiencies are due to a lack of this vitamin in the diet, a 3-month "assault plan" would include drinking a tablespoon of this yeast in some strong juice such as apple, grape or cranberry each day, and applying a once-a-week facial mask. Those who cannot tolerate or are allergic to yeast should include a high B complex vitamin supplement in their daily diet. The brewer's yeast mask sometimes brings out impurities from the system in the form of blotches, although these disappear in a short time. For this reason it is not advisable to use this facial mask just before going out to a party. The mask is made in the following way:

hot water	few drops
honey	1 teaspoon
brewer's yeast	1 tablespoon
milk	1 teaspoon
(or favorite skin oil)	
oil for face	1 teaspoon

Add a few drops of hot water to honey to liquefy it. Blend in dried brewer's yeast. Add either milk or oil to soften. Stir into thick paste. Apply oil base to face. Pat paste on face. Allow to dry for 15 to 30 minutes. Remove with cotton wool or washcloth soaked in tepid water. Use a mild astringent such as cucumber, chamomile or witch hazel extract. (See Section 13)

Peach Facial

Use a peeled blended peach plus any of above materials and/or vitamins A and D for an easy dry-skin moisturizing facial treatment.

Oatmeal Facial

Superfatted colloidal oatmeal makes a fine nourishing and bleaching facial base. To a tablespoon of oatmeal add rose water, nettle water, elder flower water or milk. Work material into a thick paste and gently pat on the neck and face. Allow the mask to dry for at least 15 minutes. Wash off with tepid water. The oatmeal creates a silken effect on the skin. Almond meal can be substituted for the oatmeal or added to the mask.

Itchy Skin

If your skin feels itchy a lot, do not lather up with soap when you bathe, but rather try cleansing with water alone. Some itchiness responds to Dove ''soap,'' which is not actually a true soap. Keep the humidity in your house high. Use a small humidifier so that you will clean it out every day. This helps to avoid spraying bacteria into the room.

Check out persistent generalized itching with your physician, as it may be due to a systemic problem or a reaction to a prescription drug or the interaction of two different drugs.

Apple cider vinegar splashdowns, or a cupful in the bath water often eliminates minor itching. Oatmeal packs, or Aveeno (prepared colloidal oatmeal) packs, compresses or in the bath water makes many allergic reactions or other itchiness disappear promptly.

Dry Skin Itching

The itching from dry and winter skin is easily overcome with simple measures. Older adults are often plagued with itchy skin because they release far less oil and less sweat than younger people. Since long-standing itching might be a symptom of a hidden problem, check unexplained, persistent itching with your doctor.

To Do	Do Not Do
Use lukewarm water	Do not use hot water on skin
Add apple cider vinegar to bathwater, or use as splash	Do not bathe every day as water and soap dry skin
Concentrate soaping on areas that need it most—under the arm, and groin and buttocks	Do not use alkaline soaps
Apply moisturizing oils while skin is still damp	Avoid lotions with alcohol
To avoid possible soap allergies, rinse clothes several times	Do not use detergents with perfumes or enzymes
When it is cold wear a hat, scarf, mask and gloves, as the wind dries the skin	

Vitamin-Lanolin Treatment

This is listed in Section 3. It is an excellent treatment and can be used daily.

Cosmetic Vinegar

Vinegar softens dry body skin and is magical with mottled dry body or leg skin. It can be used in the bath as often as needed. Read the directions in Section 14.

Exceptionally Flaky Skin

Use the lemon-water-oil spring peeler facial listed in Section 4.

Ashy Skin

Many dark or black-skinned people find their skin turns ashy in the winter time. Treat the problem as a dry-skin problem. Change your diet and add vitamins as suggested in the earlier part of this section. Add oils to your salads, drink a lot of water for internal hydration of cells and skin, and apply oils and other nourishing creams directly to the skin while it is still damp. Apple cider vinegar in the bath water and/or splashed diluted (or straight) on the face, limbs and torso will correct most skin flakiness. Avoid contact with the eyes.

Humidifiers

Unfortunately, most apartments and houses are overheated in the winter time. If you cannot regulate the heat yourself, purchase one or several small humidifiers for different rooms. These will release water back into the air. This control of excess dryness will help your family feel healthier. Excessive dryness in the air dries the membranes of the nose and creates a climate for infection. Remember you must clean each humidifier thoroughly—small ones each day, larger ones, at least once a week to avoid a buildup of bacteria. Open the windows during the wintertime! Don't live in an entirely sealed fortress without fresh air! This simple measure can make many sickly families stronger and well again.

If you have no humidifier, buy a good hand-squeezed atomizer. Fill it with distilled or boiled water, add a teaspoon of glycerine, and spray this into your nose, on your face, and into the air of your bathroom and bedroom. Evian has a great little hand spray can for moisturizing the face.

9. ROUGH SKIN

Rough Elbows

Many women neglect this area of the body and accumulate dark, ridged, sandpaper-texture elbows. It is very easy to "cure" this condition. Lemon pulp and peel have a remarkable whitening and softening effect on skin. Keep fresh lemon halves on the kitchen sink next to the soap. Give yourself a lemon swabbing every chance you get.

Oatmeal Washes

Leftover breakfast oatmeal can be used as a wash or skin paste on any roughened area. Better still is colloidal oatmeal which needs no preparation. Keep some in a little jar in the bathroom and merely add water to make into hand, face, elbow or body paste and wash. Oatmeal is wonderful for delicate and allergic skin. Also use colloidal oatmeal baths and compresses to overcome the itching of hives.

Almond Meal Paste

Rough and blotchy skin responds to the healing qualities of almonds. Use either pulverized almonds and milk, or almond meal and milk, or almond oil and honey. Pat on hands and elbows or rough spots. Allow to dry. Rinse with tepid water. Pat dry. Add pulverized peeled apple to the almonds for increased therapeutic effect.

Cider Vinegar

Cider vinegar plus water in a 1-to-8 proportion will restore the acid covering your skin craves and keep elbows and other skin areas supple and un-flaky.

White Brandy Chap Chaser

Mix 2 parts of white brandy with 1 part of rose water for a morning and night wash. The brandy gently cleanses the surface of the skin while the rose water counteracts the drying nature of the brandy and leaves the skin natural, soft and flexible.

Narcissus-Cucumber-Brandy Wash

Another old and respected chap chaser is a tablespoon of powdered cucumber roots and narcissus roots soaked in a pint of white brandy. Use as a morning or night wash.

Daisy Heads Wash to Prevent Blotching

A folk remedy to prevent blotching is an infusion of daisy heads applied to the face for 15 minutes.

Milk

Warmed milk can cure roughened skin. It can be added to pulverized almonds, cooked or colloidal oatmeal, powdered cucumber roots, powdered narcissus roots or daisy heads.

Milk Lotion

milk	½ pint
glycerine	½ ounce
bicarbonate of soda	½ ounce
borax	½ ounce

Warm the milk and slowly add glycerine, bicarbonate of soda and borax until all three dissolve. Place in labeled bottle in refrigerator. This is an excellent lotion for roughened skin.

Rose Water and Glycerine

You can buy this very healing substance in any drugstore. For a recipe see Chapter VII.

Herb Chap Chasers

Comfrey is a remarkable skin-healing herb which strengthens cell formation and helps cure rough or chapped areas. It is high in mucilage, as is also the common mallow, from which the confection marshmallow was originally made. Marigold flowers (calendula) is a good healer. Make an infusion of comfrey or marigold, or a decoction of mallow or comfrey root. Add to any hand ointment or cream, to rose water and glycerine combined, or various washes, mentioned previously. Use externally.

Eczema

Eczema is an annoying, tenacious skin problem which can emerge when one feels under stress, but the cause is basically nutritional. Some eczema patients also seem to be sensitive to milk products. It pays to do some detective work to see if there is a food connection.

A folk cure for eczema is eating one raw peeled (unsprayed) potato a day, another is eating huge amounts of fresh watercress. Homeopathic nine-grain cress tablets are prescribed by homeopaths and osteopaths for this condition. The late master-herbalist Father Kunzle recommends a wormwood tincture or infusion to help with eczema, eruptions, and scabs.

Foods high in B vitamins help eczema patients, as do B complex supplements. Use 50 mg–100 mg B complex, or nutritional brewer's yeast each day. Research indicates people with eczema may be deficient in, or lacking absorption of essential oils. This is easy to rectify either with capsules of unsaturated fatty acids, or capsules of any of the following oils: flaxseed, black currant seed, borage, evening primrose. Capsules can be taken twice daily. Child's dose is 250 mg, an adult dose is 500 mg. The results of this regimen will usually show up in about two months, after which you can cut the dose by half. To my observation, eczema patients may need this nutritional reinforcement for their entire lifetime. As a secondary effect, these oils, which incidentally act as coenzymes to B vitamins, keep the skin looking younger, and overcome and control dry or brittle hair and brittle nails.

10. THREAD VEINS

Small thread veins or broken veins on the face can respond to careful treatment and increase in vitamin C and rutin products. Rutin can be obtained from buckwheat products or tablets, while vitamin C intake can be increased with either a high-grade *natural* supplement or such foods as parsley, grapefruit, oranges or rose hips. *Don't* drink coffee, tea or alcohol, since these dilate the veins. Instead use herb teas, peppermint, chamomile and particularly coltsfoot, which is soothing internally and externally. And never use steam saunas, or facial steaming, or any hot water on the skin, only tepid water.

Coltsfoot Compresses

Coltsfoot can be used externally as well as internally as a tea. Before applying, clean your face with a mild cleanser. Pat some warm milk on your face, especially in the thread vein area. Allow to dry for 15 minutes. Wash off with soft cloth and tepid water. To make the compress, make a milk or water infusion with coltsfoot following the directions in Chapter I. Place the warm steeped herb in a cloth napkin. Apply to the veined area just after it has been washed free of the warm milk.

Yeast/Wheat Germ Mask

This mask is nourishing for the skin, and weekly applications for several months will alleviate most vein conditions.

whole egg	1 teaspoon
dried brewer's yeast	1 teaspoon
wheat germ	1 teaspoon
wheat germ oil	1 teaspoon

Blend together egg, yeast, wheat germ, wheat germ oil. Gently pat on face. Allow to dry for 15 minutes. Wash the facial off with soft cloth and tepid water. Pat face dry again. Apply a gentle coating of wheat germ oil, or any other skin nourishing oil.

Dry Skin

Many people with thread veins on their face have dry skin areas which need special attention. A mask of brewer's yeast and wheat germ, followed by wheat germ oiling of the area, should help with this condition. Another effective food combination is a green pepper and honey mask. Liquidize half a small pepper and add a tablespoon of honey. After the face is thoroughly cleansed, dab it with the inner rind of orange, lemon or grapefruit. Then add the mask. For other remedies for dry skin, see Section 8.

Oily Skin

The herbs and foods suggested in Section 6 will help to control the excessive secretion of oil to the skin. The following mask should also help.

Make a mixture of parsley juice and honey and pat over the face. For particularly oily skin add also several drops of either lemon juice or cider vinegar to the mask. Dry on face for 15 minutes. Remove later with tepid water.

Marigold (Calendula) Lotion or Ointment

One herbally important variety of marigold is known officially as calendula. Calendula leaves and flowers are both used in notable remedies. To assemble a wash for thread veins: steep calendula leaves in boiling water for 20 minutes to 3 hours. Strain. Pat the tepid liquid on face. Keep on as long as it is comfortable, then gently wash off. One can easily purchase reliable ointments made of calendula. All are exceptionally healing for the skin. Weleda makes excellent calendula products for children. Other calendula products are manufactured by homeopathic pharmacies.

11. DOUBLE CHIN

The chin, neck and jawline are often the first areas of the face to sag. The reasons are lack of circulation in jawline, lack of sufficient protein and possibly raw vegetables in the diet, and/ or depletion of vitamin E, which often shows up among women approaching the menopause. In general, it is better to start vitamin E therapy in small doses and work slowly upward.

This vitamin is widely distributed in plants and animal tissue. Particularly rich sources are green leaves, and oil from cereal seeds, especially wheat germ oil, and the vegetable oils soy bean, corn, and peanut in that order. Dairy products like milk, butter, eggs have vitamin E, as do liver, various fruits and brown rice, barley, rye, nuts, legumes. You can easily increase your daily intake of vitamin E through a diet which also includes apples, sweet corn and dried beans.

After increasing your daily intake of both protein and vitamin E, there are several daily exercises you should try.

Neck Exercises

My favorite neck exercise is the clockwise and counter-clock-wise *circular* motion. Do each 3 times. Try to make the motions fluid. You will find this extremely relaxing. Inhale deeply and hold breath until you return to first position.

Move the neck forward and back—the *"yes, yes"* motion. Inhale with head upright. Forward—hold—exhale. Lift up. Inhale; three times.

Move the neck from side to side—the *"no, no"* motion. Inhale deeply with head upright. Exhale with each slow side motion. Repeat 3 times.

Head push. With elbows resting on table, clasp hands at the back of the neck on the lower part of the head. Inhale. Gently press head down to chest. Exhale. Return to forward, front position. Inhale. Press head gently to right shoulder. Exhale. Return to forward position. Inhale. Press head to left shoulder. Exhale, Return. Inhale. Press head back. Exhale. Return upright. Inhale.

Double chin push. This isometric exercise will prevent a double chin, but it is an extremely difficult exercise to perfect.

With elbows resting on table, mesh fingers of both hands together in a "Here's the church" clasp and push against your chin. At the same time push your chin against your locked hands. Push equally hard on chin and hands and hold pressure for a count of 20. (You might prefer starting with a count of 5 and working up to a count of 20.) You should be very tired from the exercise.

Once you have mastered the exercises, added the foods rich in vitamin E and perhaps added a small amount of vitamin E supplement to your diet, you should experiment with the following nourishing neck massages.

Oil Treatments

There are any number of rich oils which can nourish your sensitive and dry neck area. The easiest of all would be a nightly rub of wheat germ oil massaged *upwards* from the bottom of the neck to the chin. Some people love the smell of wheat germ oil. If it doesn't appeal to you, use slightly warmed peanut or corn oil. Cocoa butter would be helpful in nightly massage, and even better than plain cocoa butter is a double-boiler version with lanolin.

Cocoa Butter Neck Smoother

cocoa butter	1 tablespoon
lanolin	1 tablespoon
wheat germ oil	½ cup
(or corn or peanut oil)	

optional

water	4 tablespoons

Melt all 3 oils in the top of a double boiler until all are completely dissolved. Adding water makes it easier to spread. Place in a labeled jar. Refrigerate. Shake before using. Cloudiness does not impair the mixture.

Brewer's Yeast Facial

brewer's yeast	1 tablespoon
wheat germ oil	1 tablespoon
egg yolk	1

Blend together. Apply gently (do not rub) over clean neck and face area. Allow to dry 15 to 20 minutes. Wash off with tepid water. Use soft washcloth or absorbent cotton wool.

Hollywood Double Chin Treatment

glycerine	1 teaspoon
Epsom salts	½ teaspoon
simple tincture of benzoin	
(or peppermint extract)	5 drops
absorbent cotton wool	5-inch pad
elastic bandage	enough to go around head and chin

Mix glycerine, epsom salts and benzoin or peppermint together. Place on pad of cotton wool. Place under chin. Tie on the elastic bandage. Use several times a week, perhaps while doing chores or watching TV.

12. SUNBATHING

It seems the Victorians were right in their admonition to stay out of the sun. We now know that sunlight is responsible for 90% of the aging of the skin. 'Tis true, the sun provides a handsome cocoa tan to fair skins, but the sun taketh away: it dehydrates, toughens and then the *coup de grâce*: it can create a Grand Canyon of wrinkles. And there is a matter of skin cancer. For instance, Australians have had a long love affair with the sun. In Australia sunbathing has been an art, a science, even an obsession. As a result of this long fixation, Australia now leads the world in cases of malignant melanoma, a skin cancer with high fatalities. In addition, the ozone depletion seems to be felt strongly on the Australian continent, so even casual outdoor activity now means hats, sun glasses, and sunblocks. People all over the world are following the intelligent Australian example. This is especially important for light-skinned, blue-eyed adults and children. Be careful of over-exposure to sunlight!

TANNING FACTS

Blotchy skin	May be lacking in vitamin C reserves
Tanning	Uses some reserves of vitamin B because the body uses this vitamin to form the tanning color melanin
Anemic people	Cannot tan well because they lack some of the B vitamins and mineral copper
Foods to eat if in the sun	Vitamin C foods such as citrus fruits, rose hips, cantaloupe, strawberries, tomatoes Vitamin B foods such as eggs, liver, lean meat, poultry, wheat germ, yeast and unrefined cereals. Also use an all-around B complex supplement or nutritional brewer's yeast to add to soups, drinks or food

Susceptibility to Sunburn

People with fair skin (and blue or green eyes) are more susceptible to sunburn than dark-skinned, dark-eyed people. Many researchers feel light-skinned people can tolerate more sun exposure if they take daily doses of 1,000 milligrams PABA (one of the B vitamins). Taking the PABA and also applying an *external sun-*

block with an SPF (sun protection factor) greater than 15 allows even delicate-skinned redheads and tow-headed blonds to surf and sunbathe. As an additional defense, everyone should wear a light-weight brimmed hat while outdoors in the summer time. A real Panama is a good investment. Many people feel impelled to indulge in winter tans from *tanning machines*. Leading dermatologists warn that such machines are dangerous, and may lead to a skin cancer in the future. So keep yourself and any children you know out of strong midmorning and midday sun, and avoid those tanning machines!

Tanning Lotions

Sesame is one of the polyunsaturated nut oils which penetrates and softens the skin, and it is the one which most fully absorbs the ultraviolet rays of the sun. It is therefore a wonderful natural tanning aid.

If you are going swimming you might decide to use the oil only, since it resists water, but the following is a better tanning lotion:

anhydrous lanolin	¼ cup
sesame oil	¼ cup
water	¾ cup

Melt lanolin in top of double boiler. Blend together immediately with sesame oil and water. Pour in a labeled jar. Refrigerate.

If you possess a nut grinder, try grinding a handful of *sesame seeds* to make seed lotion. Blend it with a drop of water. Keep in refrigerator or add a preservative such as ¼ teaspoon of ethyl alcohol or witch hazel.

Cucumbers are also a time-honored protection against the sun.

cucumber	1 small
glycerine	½ teaspoon
rose water	½ teaspoon

Peel and chop cucumber. Squeeze out juice. Mix with glycerine and rose water.

SUNBURN AIDS

Foods to be used topically	Diluted solution of apple cider vinegar and water
	Mashed pulp of cucumber
	Raw grated potato or potato juice
	Beaten egg white plus 1 teaspoon of honey and ½ teaspoon of witch hazel
	Equal parts of apple cider vinegar and olive oil
	Strong solution of ordinary tea. The tannic acid and theobromine in tea help remove heat from the sunburn.
Herbs to be used externally	Nettle or sage tea
	Witch hazel extract splashes or compresses
	Witch hazel plus olive oil and glycerine
	Aveeno (collodial oatmeal) compresses
Baths	Add apple cider vinegar to bath
	Add Aveeno to bath

Skin Whiteners—Sunburn Bleaches

You can revitalize and whiten the skin with ordinary buttermilk or yogurt, lemon and egg white, milk and lemon, potatoes, grapes and several flower waters. Remember, though, that all these are drying agents and are best used by those with oily complexions.

Make a herb mask by steeping fennel or elder flower in boiled water for an hour. Strain. Add a tablespoon of either buttermilk or yogurt for a bleaching mask.

Pomade de Seville

egg white   equal amounts
lemon juice

Beat egg and lemon together. Set over slow fire. Stir until mixture thickens. Label jar and keep in refrigerator. This is a popular Spanish sunburn bleach which I learned from the wife of a bull ranch owner.

Mild Bleach

lemon	1 slice
milk	½ cup

Soak lemon in milk. Strain. Pat on face and leave overnight.

Lemon Cream

sweet cream	2 teaspoons
milk	½ pint
lemon	1
brandy	3 ounces
alum powder	pinch
sugar	1 teaspoon

Combine cream and milk. Add lemon juice, brandy, alum and sugar. Simmer for 3 minutes. Skin. When cool place in labeled jar and use. Refrigerate.

Grape Lotion

Grapes are acid, but make a milder face bleach than lemon. This recipe also works, though less well, with ripe green grapes.

unripe green grapes	1 bunch
powdered alum	1 tablespoon
salt	1 teaspoon

Moisten grapes in water. Sprinkle with a mixture of powdered alum and salt. Wrap grapes in brown paper. Bake in hot ashes or slow oven for 15 minutes. Squeeze juice of grapes and wash face with the liquid. Allow to dry for 15 minutes. Wash off with tepid water. This is a very old recipe which is claimed to remove freckles, tan and/or sunburn.

13. ASTRINGENTS

Astringents contract the skin and have a topical tonic and bracing effect. Moreover, astringents reduce the greasy aftermath of skin cream cleansers, and help to *dry oily skin.* For extra zing, add a few drops of peppermint extract to any astringent application. Those with a tendency for dry skin should seldom apply astringents.

Cucumber

As far back as the 15th century cucumbers were known to be *cooling, cleansing,* and helpful in *closing* large pores. The pH of cucumber is very close to skin pH. Researchers state that cucumbers contain a substance that may act to prevent wrinkles. To use as a cleanser, peel and lather the cucumber on the face before taking a steamy warm bath, or after a steam facial.

Even better than the plain cucumber is the cooling, satiny, mashed or grated peeled cucumber plus ¼ teaspoon of honey, blended or mixed. Bottle, label and refrigerate. Home cucumber products need refrigeration.

For an infallible toner mix three important astringents, cucumber, witch hazel extract and egg white, *all of which can be used alone.* The combination of the three together creates a delightful feeling of smoothness and skin vitality:

peeled cucumber	
witch hazel	1 teaspoon
rose water	1 teaspoon
egg white	

optional

honey	¼ teaspoon
yogurt	¼ teaspoon

Mash a whole peeled cucumber. Add witch hazel, rosewater, and beaten, frothy egg white. Blend or mix with an electric mixer. Place in labeled jar in the refrigerator. The honey, while not essential, is antiseptic and helps to nourish and cleanse the skin. The yogurt is also cleansing and adds a bleaching action.

Other cucumber masks will be found in Section 4. There is a camphor-cucumber circulation and anti-pimple mask in Section 5.

Egg White

Egg white alone, or added to other ingredients, is very astringent and drying. To use, first cleanse your face, then pat on a frothy, beaten egg white. Allow to dry for 5 to 15 minutes. Wash off with tepid water.

Witch Hazel

The American Indians used poultices of boiled witch hazel twigs and barks to stop bleeding and reduce swellings from wounds. Early American pioneers followed the Indian example, and extracts of witch hazel have been available in the standard pharmacopeia. The best drugstore brand, slightly more expensive than the generic or cheap brands, is marketed under the Dickenson label. Witch hazel helps to close large or open pores. When applied in a compress on a cloth or cotton, it reduces puffiness around the eyes and face, reduces inflammations, and relieves discomfort from sunburn. Witch hazel extract can also be used as an aftershave preparation.

Witch Hazel Frappé

honey	1 teaspoon
rose water	¾ cup
witch hazel extract	¼ cup
cider vinegar	½ teaspoon
glycerine	½ teaspoon
spirits of camphor (USP)	½ teaspoon
extract of mint	teaspoon (or 5–10 drops of peppermint oil)

```
    either:
simple tincture               5 drops
   of benzoin
      or:
alum                          pinch
few drops of green vegetable coloring
```

Add honey to rose water and mix thoroughly. Blend in witch hazel, cider vinegar, glycerine, spirits of camphor, extract of mint, tincture of benzoin or pinch of alum. Add green coloring. This preparation will be cloudy-looking, but is a marvelous astringent for every day and winter-weary skin. Keep away from the eyes. Men can use it as an aftershave bracer.

Strawberry

A squashed strawberry acts as a bracing, toning facial astringent. It will reduce oiliness and help circulation.

Lady Hamilton's Strawberry Astringent Lotion

```
brandy                    ½ pint
strawberries              enough for the brandy to
                             cover additional fresh
                             berries
camphor USP               ½ ounce cake
```

Into a pint bottle pour brandy and as many strawberries as the brandy will cover. Close bottle and leave either in the sun or a warm place for a week. Strain out and save the strawberries for a dessert. Reserve the strawberry infused brandy, and add fresh strawberries into the bottle. Now add the crumbled camphor (not mothballs, but the kind you obtain from a pharmacy or botanical source) and let it stand for a few days. Again strain out the strawberries, but this time, *don't eat them.* This lotion will last indefinitely.

Herb Astringents

In addition to all of the above-mentioned foods, there are innumerable herbs with astringent qualities. Among them is the remarkable and versatile, easily obtained chamomile. One early great herbalist claims that chamomile is at least 120 times more antiseptic than sea water. Taken internally, the tea is calming and somewhat sedative, and in steam facials, chamomile is penetrating and healing. For especially oily skins, add some strained yarrow or lady's mantle tea to the steam facial. Infusions of herbs last only a few days, but will last for a much longer time if stored in a labeled jar in the refrigerator. Like witch hazel, the strained liquid tea of chamomile can be applied on cotton balls on closed eyelids as a restorative eye potion.

The kitchen herb sage also makes up well into a cooling astringent. Pour boiling water over the herb, steep, strain and apply to the face. Nettle, in addition to being a fine astringent, is a styptic (stops blood flow from cuts). Used internally, nettle juice or tea is stimulating, cleansing and purifying.

The strongest and most drying of the herb astringents is bistort root. Bayberry bark and white oak bark are mildly astringent. Barks and roots must be simmered (made into a decoction) to release their effective substances. Strain out, and use the liquid.

Long-Lasting Herbal Astringent

herb extract	1 ounce
glycerine	1 teaspoon
simple tincture of benzoin	¼ teaspoon
boric acid powder	¼ teaspoon
witch hazel extract	3 tablespoons

optional

peppermint extract	½ teaspoon

First make a herbal extract (with ethyl alcohol; See chapter I). Add glycerine, simple tincture of benzoin and boric acid powder which has previously been dissolved in the witch hazel. Add peppermint extract for extra tightening and tingling effect.

14. COSMETIC VINEGARS

Hardly anyone thinks of vinegar as almost the perfect toiletry item. It certainly doesn't evoke the same nostalgia or sense of promise as herbal remedies. Yet it is a complement to all cosmetic herb care. It has been used for thousands of years for hair and skin care, and in folk medicine.

At home we use vinegar for body toning to eliminate fatigue, for hair rinses and light complexion washes. We always use *cider vinegar,* as the malic acid from the apples is good for both the outside and the inside of the human body; cider vinegar restores the acid mantle of the skin, and it can also be combined with honey and boiling water for a drink which I have found works for many different complaints. We buy cider vinegar six bottles at a time—some goes to the bathroom for use in the bath, some goes to concoct creams, lotions and herbal ointments and to be transformed into aromatic or cosmetic vinegar, and some goes into the kitchen, since many of us start the day with this energy-giving cider vinegar and honey drink.

This preoccupation with vinegar may surprise you; I'm still rather surprised at it myself. But over the years we have learned how efficient this inexpensive grocery item can be. Vinegar softens the skin and absolutely cancels any itching from dryness. A friend who knew of my interest in ancient remedies wondered if I could recommend something for her husband, who suffered from recent itching on his body, head and face. I suggested a cup of cider vinegar in his bath water. Two days later she telephoned and said her husband felt marvelous and his skin had a completely new texture, and—blessed relief!—didn't feel itchy any more.

The same formula works on dry winter skin—you know, the kind that looks like flaky marble—and skin that's been overdried in the sun. Vinegar can also be added to hair rinses, or home protein treatments. A cider vinegar rinse helps eliminate dandruff.

The other uncanny physical effect of cider vinegar is that it relieves tiredness. Slowly massage it into the back neck, shoulders and arms, to cure body fatigue. Sometimes, after a tiring day I use this vinegar massage, then also pop into a bath with vinegar and some antifatigue herbs (see Chapter III). If this doesn't do the trick (it usually does) I take a vitamin C tablet and a calcium citrate tablet, or a tablespoon of brewer's yeast flakes or powder in a cup of hot organic soup, and in a short time afterwards feel refreshed and full of energy.

Aromatic Vinegars

Cider vinegars can be used "straight" from the bottle. If you prefer to dilute the vinegar, or wish for an aromatic vinegar, combine one part cider vinegar plus about eight parts aromatic elder flower or rose or orange *water*. Tap water can be used in a pinch. Cosmetic vinegars have a host of uses. They can cut back on oily skin, be used after hair shampooing to cut soap residue, and instantly restore the hair's acid shield. Vinegar was much used in prior centuries as a cosmetic aid.

Cosmetic vinegars can also be created by adding to a bottle of cider or white vinegar, or for a tonic, wine vinegar, such dried or fresh herbs as lavender, violet, roses, rosemary; or oils of bergamot, lavender, rosemary, peppermint, verbena, carnation, rose geranium.

Lavender vinegar is my own favorite. It has been popular for thousands of years, and is described in one old manuscript thus: "It is cooling, and if the face is washed with it, it gives a firmness to and braces the fibres of the skin when too much relaxed."

Fresh Flower Vinegar

lavender flowers*	3 tablespoons
water	½ pint
cider vinegar	1 pint

*Or any aromatic flower

Add lavender flowers to vinegar, steep for 2 weeks and add water.

Essence Vinegar

oil or essence of lavender‡	½ teaspoon
cider or white vinegar	1 pint
water	1 pint

Aromatic Tonic Vinegar

fresh rose petals*	1 ounce
white wine vinegar	¼ pint

Use a double boiler. Let rose petals and wine vinegar steep for 20 minutes in the upper half over the boiling water. Place in jar. Cover vinegar and roses with cloth or foil. Set in warm place. Steep 2 weeks. Strain petals from lotion. Place in tightly lidded jar.

15. NATURAL DEODORANTS

Clean children don't have a body odor—it is only with the onset of puberty and hormone production that perspiration starts to have a strong aroma. Chlorophyll, a natural substance in nature, being bactericidal, has a marked effect on the bacteria which cause body odor. Therefore eat foods high in chlorophyll, or supplements high in chlorophyll, to cut perspiration odor.

When the weather is hot, or when you are active, you will perspire more. Supplement your diet with B complex and niacin-rich foods such as peanuts, bran, mushrooms, and brewer's yeast.

‡Or any aromatic oil or essence
*Or any aromatic flower petals

Food Deodorants

Food deodorants are useful to allergic people and those hesitant about using aluminum-based commercial deodorants.

All green leafy vegetables and some root tops are high in chlorophyll. The most effective antiperspiration odor foods are the dark green leaves of lettuce, parsley and the tops of beets, radish and turnip. Those who are on a vegetarian diet find they may perspire as much as they once did eating meat, but they don't have as strong a perspiration odor.

Herb, Oil, Flower Deodorants

Several herbs, oils and flowers can be helpful in controlling body odor. Sage, lovage, cleavers, leaves of chrysanthemum, and oils of lavender, camphor and pathchouli were considered outstanding deodorant aids by herbalists of prior generations.

A strong infusion of sage is used by the Chinese to control perspiration odor. Lovage and cleavers are also used in tea form as a drink, in the bath, and under the armpits.

Lavender oil is an effective natural deodorant, but it is far too strong to use as an oil, except a drop at a time as a perfume. Make up a lavender *water* following the directions in Chapter X. It makes a delightful eau de cologne, and should be on everyone's shelf.

Another antiperspirant drink that has a valued reputation is one made of oil of camphor (USP), lemon and milk. Soak some lemon peel and fruit in warm milk and add 3 drops of camphor oil to the milk. Before retiring each night you can either drink the milk or chew the lemon rind.

Two young girls I know, who were allergic to every commercial deodorant they tried, used cider vinegar plus water and reported that it was a very effective deodorant. The vinegar restores the skin to its normal pH value with its proper acid mantle, and although you still perspire there is far less odor. This treatment gets better as you use it. The smell of cider vinegar evaporates in about 10 minutes. See Section 14.

CHAPTER III

BATHING

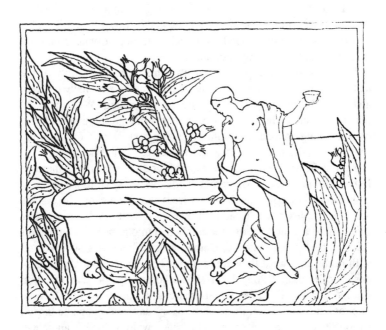

Many ancient cultures developed their social life and institutions around the idea of group bathing, and indeed the Japanese still have a form of family bathing. The ancient Assyrians restricted certain helpful herbs and oils to the royal family, and others to the nobles, while the less efficacious herbs were assigned to the common people. On the other hand, in Syria the king sometimes joined his subjects in the bathhouse. Antiochus was once accosted by one of his subjects while bathing, with the words, "You must be a happy man, O King: you smell in a most *costly* manner!" Antiochus, far from being displeased, smilingly poured his expensive unguent over the man's head, while other poorer people crowded round to capture droplets of the precious oil. The Romans also went en masse to their elegant and beautiful marble bathhouses. In the famous Baths of Caracalla, considered the most beautiful of all the ancient bathhouses, up to 2,300 Roman citizens could choose from at least two dozen highly imaginative healthy and skin-restoring mineral, steam, massage, friction or oil baths, and often rich Romans vied with each other to see whose bath oil had the most interesting fragrance.

What has to be accepted in our own time is the versatility of the bath, for it is *not* just for cleansing. A bath can be extremely relaxing and soporific, or energizing and circulation-building. With the addition of certain herbs it can be soothing, healing, calming, reviving or stimulating. A bath can soften the skin and keep it from getting rough or brittle; it can replace lost moisture, oil and acidity.

Although we owe a deep debt of gratitude to the American Indian for his system of herbal medicine—a system we are just beginning to discover again—it is from the Europeans, the Asians and the peoples of the Near East that we inherit our bath cosmetic lore. There are dozens of stories about famous beauties and their favorite herbs: for instance, Catherine the Great was so involved with herbs, and what they could do for her beauty, that she created her own Russian "Pony Express," whose only job was to comb Europe and the Far East for aromatic and skin-nourishing plants. She took a long bath in these herbs every day, and once she tarried so long that she kept a great ambassador waiting for his audience. He was so outraged that it almost caused an international incident.

The French beauty Madame de Pompadour was the mistress of Louis XV of France and from the age of twenty-four until her death virtually ruled France. She was a friend of Voltaire and other authors of the *Encyclopédie,* and employed many artists to decorate her seven châteaux. However, La Pompadour was justifiably unpopular for her extravagance, which included a complete corps—almost an army—which did nothing but search for and collect herbs for her famous baths. Because bathing had fallen into disrepute during the Middle Ages and was not yet completely in favor, Louis XV asked his physicians to entreat his mistress not to take so many baths, fearing they would destroy her beauty, but La Pompadour ignored their advice and, it is said, used her herbs to great advantage.

Nowadays you don't need an army to gather and prepare herbs, for that has been done for you by the great botanical houses. In fact, you need only to call or send a postcard for a catalogue and the world's exotic natural substances are immediately available.

Basic Needs for Bathing

Although hot water is needed initially to release the essences and principles of the herbs, oils and foods suggested here, you should never bathe in very hot water for a long time, as this de-energizes the body. Hot water is inadvisable for those with either sensitive, thin skins or thread veins on face or body.

For totally relaxing and soaking baths you should have a stretch-out tub; a non-slip mat or pasted non-slip strips, a large, comfortable rubber pillow to rest your head; and large, rough, absorbent towels.

On the subject of towels, there is some interesting advice from an outstanding hydrotherapy expert, the nineteenth-century herbalist, Father Kneipp. He suggested *not* using a towel but rather wrapping oneself into a rough cloth mantle or cotton robe, or immediately climbing into absorbent clothes and walking around or exercising until the body returned to its normal temperature.

To Read or Not to Read in the Bath

This must depend on your state of tiredness or your need to re-energize. If you want a truly relaxing bath, use the time to rest your eyes. An actress I know works very hard when she is in a film or on the stage and uses her bath time to recharge. "I turn out all the lights except a small night light, allow some more warm water to flow into the bath, and in 15 minutes I feel revitalized," she says. "I find cucumber slices restful for my eyes, so while bathing, I often place one on each eye, and gently palm each piece until the juice clears the eyes."

16. HERB BATHS

How to Use Herbs in the Bath

The one thing you must not do is just throw herbs *into* the bath. The smell is marvelous and they have a therapeutic effect of course; but if you try it, you will discover it takes about an hour to dislodge all the pieces of leaves, berries or bark from your body. So the thing to do is to use either a bath pochette or a strong herb infusion. Directions for infusion can be found in Chapter I.

You can make a bath pochette by enclosing your favorite herbs in a bag made of porous cloth, such as cheesecloth. For a more attractive effect, put the disposable cheesecloth bag in a patterned or colorful muslin or silk drawstring bag. These can be hung over the hot water tap and used for many consecutive baths. A modern version which works well for me is one of those oval, stainless steel hinged tea containers for making individual cups of tea. Most of them have chains, and some can be tied to the hot water tap, or allowed to float freely in the bathtub.

Two Versatile Herbs

Chamomile is a mild apple-smelling yellow and white flower. it is one of the most versatile of all herbs, and can be used in hair rinses, hair dyes, eye washes, facials. It contains azulene, a most soothing substance to the skin. Use the fresh leaves and flowers, or the dried flowers.

Since chamomile makes an excellent cleansing substance, it is good for body care in the bath. For an extra fillip and a more stimulating action use ½ cup of chamomile with a dash of rosemary, horsetail and pine needles (or extract). During the summer when you are plagued by insect bites, chamomile will protect you. Use in the bath; afterwards pat on a strong infusion of the flowers over all exposed parts of the body, and most insects will avoid you.

Elder leaves, berries, bark and flowers are considered healing for eyes; as an ointment, healing for sores of all kinds; and in infusion soothing for the nerves and helpful in falling asleep. In the bath elder can bleach, heal and stimulate the skin.

Aromatic Herbs

Every period of history has had its own attitude toward bathing. In England in the 17th century perfumed baths came into favor, and roses, lemon flowers, jasmine, bay, lavender, mint, pennyroyal and citron peel were used alone or together with a few drops of oil of spike and some fixative such as musk or ambergris. It is quite simple to obtain these oils and essences today, and you can certainly combine them for your aromatic baths.

Lovage, a member of the parsley family, is not a highly aromatic herb, but it has the virtue of being cleansing, refreshing and deodorant. Gently boil the lovage root for 20 minutes. Strain and use. For more on natural deodorants, see Section 15.

Healing Herbs

There are many healing herbs, but not all lend themselves to infusion and use in the bath. Of the several that I would recommend, *comfrey* has the extraordinary power to help mend fractured bones. Country folk call it "knit-bone." The leaves can make a valuable poultice for all kinds of sores, burns, swellings, and can be used in strong infusion in the bath water. The roots, too, release a large amount of mucilage, which is easily extracted by hot water.

Lady's mantle, a delightful pleated herb (hence the name), is valued by the Arabs for all kinds of women's troubles. Externally it can help heal inflammations and even acne.

Marigold (calendula) leaves also have a reputation for healing, and are available in ointment form. The leaves can be used in tepid baths to help those with body scars, thread veins and soothing varicose veins.

The Latin name for yarrow is *Achillea millefolium.* The herb is a useful and powerful astringent, and therefore is of special interest to those with excess oil on their face and body since it can be used in the bath, in an infusion as a facial ingredient, and internally as a tea. When used as a tea it can bring on perspiration and thus cleanse the system.* If you feel an illness coming on, drink a strong infusion with equal parts of yarrow, peppermint and elder flower. Hop into bed and go to sleep. You will feel much better when you awaken. A yarrow compress can also alleviate soreness of the nipples.

Linden (lime) and *nettle* leaves contain a compound physiologically related to natural hormones, and are helpful for body skin. In addition, nettles contain the vitamins A and C. *Dandelions* also have many plant hormones and can be combined with nettles for a most cleansing and helpful bath.

Mint has healing properties and can be used in the bath to heal minor skin eruptions.

Houseleek has always been considered a valuable skin herb, and can be used for healing and nourishing baths.

The famous French beauty Ninon de Lenclos, who remained unwrinkled and youthful-looking to a great old age, was exceptionally fond of houseleek in her creams and facials. It is said that her secret bath herbs were a combination of houseleek, mint, lavender, thyme and rosemary.

Nourishing Baths

Most women use creams and nourishing products on the face. However, a large majority of women forget to apply restorative massage creams and body oils to soothe, soften and replenish the rest of their body. Almond and avocado oil are highly nourishing for the body. However, less expensive salad oils such as sunflower, sesame seed and peanut oils, are available from supermarket shelves, and can be used on the skin.

Herbal Bath Oils

Dispersing oil is one that completely dissolves in water. There are very few of these, but the oil of the castor plant can, when treated, be an ideal bath oil, as it dissolves completely and does not leave a ring. Treated castor oil is known as Turkey-red oil.

---

*Avoid if pregnant.

| Turkey-red oil | ¾ cup |
| aromatic oil | ¼ cup |

Mix together. Bottle. Label. Use 1 teaspoon per bath.

Floating oil is one that is lighter than water and floats on top. It will cling to your skin as you emerge from the bath. Almond oil and avocado oil are such oils.

almond oil	¾ cup
aromatic oil	¼ cup
or, an alternative recipe	
almond oil	½ cup
avocado oil	¼ cup
aromatic oil	¼ cup

Mix together. Bottle. Label. Use 1 teaspoon per bath.

Any of these oils will cost far less and be far purer than most commercially available bath capsules. With a little experimentation, particularly with different scents, you should be able to make up bath oils for yourself and your family, and as gifts for friends.

Herbal Oil Soap

chamomile	2 tablespoons
(or nettle, lime flower, elder flower, fennel)	
milk	12 tablespoons
egg	1
almond oil	8 tablespoons
herbal shampoo	2 tablespoons
honey	1 teaspoon
(or coconut oil shampoo or castile shampoo)	
isopropyl alcohol	2 tablespoons
(or perfume)	

Drench chamomile (or other suggested herb) in the cold milk and let it stand with a porous cover for 3 hours. Strain. Discard chamomile flowers. Put herb-milk aside. Mix the egg with the almond oil and beat until entirely smooth. Add and keep mixing the shampoo, and as you keep beating also add the honey and isopropyl rubbing alcohol. Blend in the herb-milk. Pour into a labeled jar. This needs frequent shaking, but is a useful and effective bath oil soap. Should you decide to take it up in larger quantities, keep it in the refrigerator.

For a more aromatic effect, cut oil to 6 tablespoons and add combination of 1 tablespoon oil of lavender, ½ tablespoon of oil of lemon, ¼ tablespoon of oil of cloves.

For increased stimulation from this bath oil soap, particularly in the case of body aches, add ¼ teaspoon of either oil of pine or oil of eucalyptus to the original recipe.

17. SOOTHING AND TONING BATHS

Oatmeal, Almond Meal, Cornmeal, Bran Baths

When I was about ten a remarkable woman moved into our house as our housekeeper. I adored the septuagenarian Mrs. Nox. One of the things she taught me was never to throw away leftover oatmeal. She showed me how to use it in my nightly bath. Oatmeal is soothing, and cleansing, and keeps the body milky-white. It also heals inflamed skin.

Good pharmacies all carry a superfatted colloidal oatmeal under the brand name Aveeno. Since it is rather expensive, you may want to use it only on special occasions or when the skin feels itchy, or when someone has an allergic reaction like hives. To use, plaster a dampened handful over the body, or an affected itchy or sensitive part of the body, and throw another handful into the bath water too. Remove the body "mask" with a soft washcloth or a softened sponge. I always keep some Aveeno in a pretty container in the bathroom for emergencies.

Almond meal has almost the same soothing effect as oatmeal. Cornmeal or branmeal are also useful. It is harder to disperse these last powders in the bath water. But you can blend the meals, or grind them in a food processor. The smaller the particles the better.

Milk Baths

Many beauties of the past, including Cleopatra, were known for their extravagant milk baths. Milk is an extremely nourishing, soothing substance and will help smooth the skin and give it a lustrous finish. It is healing for roughened skin. Tepid milk baths (or facials) are helpful both for acne and for blackheads (see Section 5).

For additional softening power in a milk bath, add a strong infusion of elder flower or chamomile, or nettle, or lime flower (linden).

George Sand's Replenishing Milk Bath

When the Baroness Aurore Dudevant left her husband and went to live and work with the writer Jules Sandeau, she changed her name to George Sand. She earned her living, and supported her children, by writing; some of her eighty novels are certainly autobiographical, and describe her liaisons with, among others, the poet Alfred de Musset and the composer Chopin. The truth is that George Sand wasn't a great beauty. But in addition to talent, brains and charm, she had a lovely, alive-looking, youthful skin which she smartly took pains to preserve. Her secret was the use of lots of farm milk and honey and salt and her era's version of bicarbonate of soda in her baths. She knew that salt removes toxins and dead skin cells, and the honey and milk and bicarbonate of soda are skin softeners. A modern, scaled-down George Sand bath would be: dissolve into a glass of warm milk a handful of coarse salt, two tablespoons of honey, and (optional) a tablespoon or two of bicarbonate of soda. Pour into bath just as you are getting into it.

Expensive Baths

There were several famous beauties who had nightly baths in berries—some used strawberries, others raspberries. Isabelle of Bavaria took spring and summer baths in strawberry juice. Strawberries, of course, are delightfully cooling and cleansing to the skin, and they have internal cleansing power too. Another famous beauty, Madame Tallien, favored a bath of crushed strawberries and raspberries, after which she was gently rubbed with sponges soaked in perfumed milk. Mary Queen of Scots preserved her beauty by bathing in wine, a habit which the Earl of Shrewsbury, in whose charge she was, found so costly that he had to ask the government to increase his allowance for taking care of the queen.

Tonic Spring Baths

Everyone who lives in a cold winter climate longs for a tonic bath to brighten dingy winter skin. If you are lucky enough to know where there are unsprayed blackberry leaves, collect and crush them and add boiling water to make an especially strong infusion. These blackberry leaves are particularly effective if used several nights in a row in your bath water. Your skin will have a new look and glow.

Friction Baths

The body is constantly renewing its cells and actually replaces all of them in a seven-year period. Wherever you increase your circulation with exercise, toweling, salt, oil or loofah or brush rubs, you are aiding the process of replacement, and you will look and feel far better.

Circulation Baths

The famous mineral and ocean spas provide excellent circulation baths. It is hard to obtain the special mineral mud from mineral spas, but you will find it quite simple to make your own circulation bath. Combine ½ pound of magnesium sulphate (Epsom salts) and 1 pound of coarse salt in your warm bath. If you want to have a health-giving touch and an invigorative smell, add eucalyptus, pine or mint extract or oil. If you want to use your own pine needles, either boil them for 20 minutes or place them in a large Thermos flask, pour boiling water over them, let them steep for 12 to 24 hours, and strain and use a cupful at a time.

Salt Toner Rub

Overcome sluggishness and restore body tone with a coarse salt massage and bath. I find it a never-fail energy reviver. Coarse salt is available in food markets under the Diamond brand. Use the salt either dry from the box or slightly moistened. Rub, half a handful at a time, over the shoulders and arms, and then over the rest of the body, omitting the groin area and the face (although tiny amounts of *saltwater* can be *sniffed up the nostrils* at this time to clear nasal passages). Hot baths are relaxing, but hot water also depletes one's energy. For an energizing bath, immerse yourself in warm water, and end a bath or shower with a cold water splash, especially to the feet. To further restore yourself—*do not dry yourself,* instead wrap your wet body in a bath sheet, and hop into bed under covers for an instant and remedial 15-minute nap. Or if you are going right to sleep, discard the cumbersome towel after a few minutes—you'll feel warm and toasty, and ready for a long peaceful, quiet sleep session.

Detoxifying Bath: Epsom salts, magnesium sulphate, produces perspiration which releases impurities through your pores. Add a handful of Epsom salts to a warm (not too hot) bath, and soak until you perspire. Because the Epsom salts' detoxifying action causes lassitude, go right to bed afterwards and try to fall asleep. Do not use this bath if you are pregnant or have any circulation or heart condition.

Cider Vinegar Bath or Rub

A cup of apple cider vinegar provides an instant antifatigue bath which also restores the skin's acid mantle covering. Apple cider vinegar takes away any itchiness, flakiness and dryness of the skin.

Toning Baths

There is nothing like water for toning up the body. For an immediate refreshing pickup, try the *cold friction bath.* For only a few seconds or minutes, depending on your tolerance to the cold, dip your body into inches of cold water, all the time rubbing your body with a rough washcloth, or a loofah, a softened vegetable sponge. Once out of the bath, either towel yourself dry, or get into absorbent clothes such as a sweat suit and exercise until you feel warm. You'll feel marvelous afterwards.

For general everyday toning up of the body, and an immune booster, try frequent *cold water foot baths.* Stand in the cold running water in your bathtub for seconds to minutes either up to your ankles, or up to your calves. This can be done first thing every morning, and the last thing every night.

Cold knee bath dunks. These are refreshing and stimulating to the entire body, and can be used first thing in the morning, or just before going to bed, to induce sleep. The best way to do this is to run about 5 or 6 inches of cold water in the bath, and kneel in the water for a few seconds to a few minutes.

Alternate hot and cold foot baths, or an alternate hot and cold shower to the feet acts to tone the body, and helps to overcome a feeling of great fatigue. The effect of this shower can be increased by standing under a warm shower, and having a cold hand shower attached to the bath faucet, and spraying the area with cold water at the same time. End with cool to cold water.

CHAPTER IV

HAIR

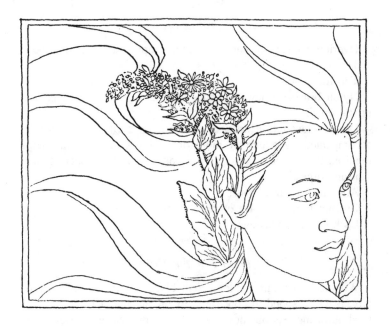

Hair is a fairly good indicator of general health, as are the complexion, clearness of the eyes and color and quality of the fingernails. It is one of the doctor's instant indicators of negative or positive health.

Like the outer covering on our body and fingernails, hair is a form of skin—a protein, actually—called keratin. It gets its nourishment from the food we eat, and therefore fairly quickly indicates either the lack of nutrients, or often, the lack of absorption of specific foods. Most adults have about 100,000 hairs growing on their heads, and these can survive for between two years and ten, depending on age, race and sex.

If you have the right genes—if your grandparents and parents had strong hair—you will too. The other factors that affect healthy hair are stress, and sleep, and adequate protein. Also, your hair needs an internal source of oil and moisture.

Hair Enemies

Overindulgence in carbohydrates, empty dry cereals, cake, soda, sugar.

Too much sun.

Nylon brushes (they split ends and damage hair). Use natural bristle brush.

Drugs. Prescription drugs in the form of antibiotics should be accompanied by a cup or more of yogurt a day, as this helps replaced the "good" bacteria your body needs for proper absorption and digestion.

Allergies and infection.

Chemicals in the form of rinses, tints and bleaches.

Lack of scalp massage.

Food For the Hair

Whether your hair is blond, red, black or brown, dull, dry or oily, it will respond to consistent, intelligent internal and external food nurturing. Serious or chronic illness, or lack of the right food can strongly influence hair texture by slowly removing nutrients from the hair, as well as the nails, teeth and skin. The body does this to feed and protect the more important internal organs. The B complex vitamins, especially pantothenic acid (B5), B6, and inositol and niacin (B3) are critical for hair vitality and growth. Unsaturated fatty acids such as black currant oil, borage, evening primrose or flaxseed, are necessary for a vigorous, strong texture, and to prevent dry, or brittle hair. Vitamin C is important for the entire immune operation, and to provide improved scalp activity.

Vitamin E has many functions: it contributes to oxygen intake, and supports increased scalp vigor. Zinc prompts hair growth by augmenting immune performance (small amounts of copper chelate in your multivitamin helps the zinc to do its job). Kelp supplies iodine, which stimulates the thyroid gland to maintain essential scalp energy. Coenzyme Q10 augments tissue oxygenation and scalp circulation.

For graying hair, take PABA tablets. To enhance hair growth take small amounts of L-cysteine and L-methionine.

Important foods for hair restoration are green salads and fresh raw vegetables, particularly watercress, white part of leeks, carrots and potatoes, and such fruits as apples and oranges. Fresh fish and some sea vegetation, organic liver once or twice a week, raisins and monounsaturated olive oil, or polyunsaturated oils such as safflower, sunflower, soy, wheat germ, corn, or capsules of any of the omega-rich oils such as evening primrose, flaxseed, black currant or borage are important parts of a hair restoration diet.

18. SCALP EXERCISES

The best way to increase the circulation of your scalp is to learn the yoga headstand and do it every day. If this is too difficult, the next best thing is the preparatory posture—the shoulder stand, which is much easier. Lie on your back, then raise your body and rest it on your shoulders and elbows. Keep your feet high and legs straight. You will feel the chest pressing on the neck and the thyroid gland, and this helps to activate it. Daily rest or exercise on a slant board increases circulation in the scalp.

The following is a head massage which you can practice any time of the day.

Curl up each hand as though you were grasping a rather slippery orange, so that your fingers are tensed and strong. With the cushion of each of your ten tensed fingers, press down in a circular motion until you feel the warmth of the blood rushing to the area. Then move on to another spot on the scalp until your whole head is tingling and alive. Push and tug, rub, stroke, tap, drum, massage and knead your scalp as you awaken each day. This will give you a feeling of well-being and vitality, and eventually will increase scalp circulation.

19. SHAMPOOING

When you feel unwell, even if you have a cold, it helps to shampoo and massage your scalp. This touching of vital trigger and *chi* energy points acts to start an internal healing process.

Make a herbal shampoo by adding a strong infusion of herbs to your favorite coconut, castile or avocado shampoo. Also, you can add these herbs to a plant substance containing nature's soaping ingredient—saponin.

For a *light hair* shampoo, make a strong chamomile infusion and add to shampoo. Besides being a hair lightener, chamomile is a softening agent.

Add an infusion of mullein flowers or nettle, or a decoction of rhubarb root.

Those with normal or oily light hair can add a beaten egg white; those with dry light hair a beaten egg yolk.

For a *dark hair* shampoo, add either rosemary or sage infusion, or rosemary oil. These herbs revitalize hair.

Dry Shampooing

In many parts of the world, particularly the Far East where the women and men pride themselves on their long, lustrous and healthy hair, few people ever *wash* the hair. Instead they brush through it some form of absorbent meal or powder, depending on available resources. In India, for instance, those who follow the old ways use a form of cornmeal and brush it through the hair until it is clean. The advantage of these dry shampoos is the sparkling look they give to the hair once it is properly brushed out, and the boost the hair gets when its necessary 2 per cent acid mantle is not constantly washed out.

Orrisroot from pulverized Florentine iris root has been used for dry shampoos for many centuries. Fuller's earth can also be used.

Part the hair in sections and sprinkle in the absorbent substance until the whole head has been covered at the scalp. Brush vigorously 5 minutes later.

I learned of this dry shampoo from a film makeup man who used it when working under difficult location shooting. When there is no time or place to wash a head of hair he covers a hairbrush with a piece of cheesecloth or nylon stocking, and forces the fabric through the brush bristles. He sprinkles this with eau de cologne, and brushes through the hair. A surprising amount of dust and grey dirt will adhere to the cloth. The cloth can be thrown away and the same process repeated again if there is more dirt in the hair.

20. CONDITIONERS

If you are not endowed with lustrous hair by family inheritance, you need a conditioner. To condition hair properly, wash it first with herbal shampoo. Add conditioner-treatment. Allow time for it to "take." Rinse out the conditioner. Set or dry the hair.

Hot Oil

A topical hot oil treatment adds luster, even brilliance to the hair. Penetrating and effective hair oils are (in order of importance) olive oil, almond oil, avocado oil, safflower and corn oil. You can use a hot oil treatment once a week.

Heat the oil and saturate the hair. Cover the hair with a layer of wax paper or plastic wrap. Cover hair again with a heavy-duty plastic cap. Add heat with a towel-wrap. In times past I thought there was nothing better than adding heat with an electric cap, but now we know that there are consequences in electromagnetic waves, especially close to the body or the head.* If you wrap the head well, you can leave the oil on throughout the night. When you wash out the oil, the hair will glisten and feel more supple.

*Keep electromagnetic forces away from your body. Do not use an electric blanket, or an electric heat pad (instead use a hot water bottle). Get rid of digital clocks, if they are at the head or side of your bed, and buy a battery clock instead. Stand at least 3 feet away from active microwave ovens.

Protein Treatments

Eggs contain an excellent hair-helping protein and lecithin, a substance which restores hair texture and luster. The following are two protein treatments which include eggs. First wash the hair. Apply treatment and let it seep into hair for 15 minutes to 30 minutes. Rinse out.

Protein Cure

The following treatment combines protein, emollients and lecithin, all of which are helpful to brittle hair:

lanolin	3 tablespoons
castor oil	3 tablespoons
olive oil	¼ cup
liquid castile soap	1 tablespoon
glycerine	4 tablespoons
water	1¼ cups
egg yolk	2 tablespoons
cider vinegar	1 teaspoon
eggs	2

In the top of a double boiler blend together lanolin, castor oil and olive oil. Turn off the heat for at least 5 minutes and let the blended oils sit. Slowly, with an electric mixer, stir in liquid castile soap, glycerine and water. Use a low speed until the mixture thickens. With the beater on high add 2 tablespoons of beaten egg yolk and cider vinegar. Pour into a jar, label and refrigerate for several hours or overnight. Next add 2 whole eggs on high speed. After applying protein treatment, store leftovers in refrigerator for later use.

Quick Protein Cure

eggs	1 or 2 (depending on hair brittleness)

castor oil	1 tablespoon
(or wheat germ, olive, corn, safflower oil)	
glycerine	1 tablespoon
cider vinegar	1 teaspoon

Beat together all ingredients. Apply after initial shampoo. Leave on for at least 15 minutes to ½ hour. Rinse.

For instant relief use a good store-bought mayonnaise.

Cocoa Butter Conditioner

The hair is happy with the cocoa butter recipe used for dry skin cleansing. Here safflower oil stretches out the recipe.

safflower oil	½ cup
cocoa butter	1 tablespoon
anhydrous lanolin	1 tablespoon

In the top of a double boiler melt together the oil, the cocoa butter and the lanolin until they are *completely* dissolved and blended together. Beat with an electric mixer. Take about 3 tablespoons of above mixture and add 1 tablespoon of water. Mix again. Label the jar as cocoa butter conditioner. Use on hair if it is very dry.

Parsnip Conditioner

This is vouched for by a lady whose great-great-grandmother passed it on to her.

Simmer together 1 chopped parsnip root, ½ teaspoon of parsnip seeds and ¼ cup of olive oil (or *any* of the previously mentioned oils). Steep for ½ hour. Strain and use on hair.

21. DRY HAIR

Sometimes people aren't sure whether their hair is normal or dry. Two good tests are how it looks and feels to the touch. Does your hair look bright and have luster? Does it shine and glisten when just washed? Does it feel dry and/or brittle to the touch? If you have answered no to the first two questions and yes to the last question, you have dry hair. If you have dry hair without much vitality and bounce, make a determined effort to eliminate sugar and sugar products from your diet. Sugar depletes and destroys your B complex vitamins, and you need these vitamins for radiant hair and skin.

Shampooing Dry Hair

Do not shampoo dry hair too often. In summer, once a week is best. First wash your hair with a restorative herbal shampoo. (If it is especially limp add a whole beaten egg, or preferably 2 egg yolks and ½ packet of unflavored gelatine dissolved in ¼ cup of boiling water.) Condition your hair—see Section 20. Rinse out the conditioner.

Condition the hair *after* you wash it, and just rinse out the conditioner. In this way you do not neutralize or cancel out the effects of the conditioner.

Restoring Luster

Rosemary is particularly effective for people with dark hair. Oil of rosemary untangles hard-to-manage hair and adds sheen.

rosemary	2 tablespoons
boiling water	1 pint
oil of sweet almonds	3 ounces
lavender essence	10 drops

Mix together 1 ounce of an infusion of rosemary and almond oil and lavender to create a scented luster-restorer for dark hair.

Parsley can also be used. Boil it in water for 20 minutes. Use water as a final rinse to add sheen to hair.

22. OILY HAIR

Although oily hair seems harder to manage than dry hair, it can be brought back to normal with proper diet, consistent and careful brushing, scalp massage and exercise. Excess oil in the hair means that the sebaceous glands of your scalp are far too active, and you should immediately cut down on animal fats and fried foods in your diet. Occasionally, too, oily hair is a result of poor thyroid function and stress. If you suspect either, you should see your doctor.

Antistrain Relaxer

One exercise which stimulates the thyroid is the following antistrain relaxer, which increases the circulation to your shoulders and neck:

Lie on your back with your palms up and rest for a few minutes. Close your eyes. Your body should feel heavy. Clench your left hand. Lift it, tense it hard. Let it fall limply so that all tension disappears. Do this for your right hand. Lift and tense your left leg, then let it fall limply. Same for the other leg. Then grimace. Make a tense, sour face. Stick out your tongue, push out your eyes. Let your face relax. Starting with your toes and concentrating on each part of your body, force yourself to relax until you are completely limp and relaxed. Lie like this for as long as you wish.

Then *lift your head* up until your chin is resting on your neck. Do this several times. This encourages thyroid activity. So does the *shoulder stand.* Lift your entire body up until it rests on your elbows and feel the pressure of the thyroid on the chest. This exercise is excellent for everybody and will help revitalize hair and skin, and will help you look younger and vital.

Food for Oily Hair

Foods rich in iodine and food with high B complex factors are helpful in eliminating oily hair. Soybeans, soy sauce, seaweed and kelp are also helpful. Drink yarrow or lady's mantle tea. Add yarrow infusion to your shampoo. Use frequent cider vinegar rinses after shampoo—½ cup to a quart of water.

Oily Hair Shampoos

Shampoo oily hair often, even once a day.

Dark-haired people with oily hair can use any of the following herbs added to castile or other herbal shampoos.

Make a decoction of 1 tablespoon of southernwood, 1 tablespoon of quassia chips. Simmer together in 1 pint of water for 20 minutes. Add a teaspoon of rosemary. Steep for another 3 minutes. Cool. Strain and add to shampoo.

Another drying shampoo which also restores luster and body to the hair is the following:

whole eggs	2
rum	¼ cup
rose water	¼ cup

Beat eggs and massage through hair. Wash off 15 minutes later. Rinse with equal parts of rum and rose water.

If you can't wash your hair every day, an orrisroot, or fuller's earth *dry* shampoo is very effective, as is the nylon- or cheese-cloth-covered hair brush to remove dirt and grime. Oily hair responds to vigorous and constant brushing.

23. FINAL RINSES

Vinegar

Diluted cider vinegar rinses have been used for centuries. Vinegar restores the acid covering that has been washed away with shampoo. It also removes the last vestiges of soap in the hair. (See Section 14).

Dark Hair Rinses

Add two teaspoons of blueberry juice to a quart of hot water. Cool for a bit, and rinse through the hair to bring out the blue tone in truly black hair.

The kitchen herb rosemary is an excellent rinse addition for dark hair. Use 2 tablespoons to a pint of boiling water. Steep and strain. Add to final rinse water.

A herbal rinse to add luster to dark hair includes southernwood and quassia chips boiled gently for 15 minutes. Use 1 teaspoon of southernwood to 2 tablespoons of quassia chips to a pint of water. Steep for ½ hour, strain and rinse to bring out the natural highlights of dark hair. The chips are available from botanical sources.

Light Hair Rinse

You can add stunning highlights to blond and light brown hair by adding either strained chamomile infusion, or rhubarb root concoction (soup) to rinse water. The rhubarb root tends to be sticky, so use it only if you intend to rinse your hair again. Strained lemon juice, and diluted cider vinegar are also lighteners of light hair. See Section 28.

24. NATURAL SETTING LOTIONS

There are a great many natural substances which can easily be added to shampoos and rinses, or which can be used as a *setting lotion* for hair which hangs too limp and straight. While it is true these home products take a bit more time to make than shop items, they give a boost to the hair and do not leave any dry, flaky residue.

Rosemary

Rosemary is one of the best herbs for the hair and can be used in massages, rinses and shampoos as well as setting lotions.

According to Dr. Fernie, the author of the century-old *Herbal Simples*, you could do no better than wash or rinse your hair in rosemary. He recommends it particularly for rainy days. "It has the singular power," he writes, "of preventing the hair from *uncurling* when exposed to a damp atmosphere." Fernie's recipe consists of an infusion of rosemary—2 tablespoons or 1 ounce to a pint of boiling water. Steep for a few hours, strain and use either in shampoo or final rinse water.

Another version of this tonic is rosemary and equal parts of sage combined. Prepare the same way as above. Both these herbs are best for people with dark brown or black hair.

Quince, Flaxseed, Irish Moss and Gums

Nature has provided us with many natural setting lotions. Quince seed is one of the very best. Simmer a teaspoon in boiling water until the mixture thickens. For a longer-lasting quince seed setting lotion, add a tablespoon of eau de cologne to each tablespoon of dissolved seed. Quince is also a known hair reviver.

Flaxseed (linseed) and Irish moss (carragheen) also add body to the hair. To use either one, dissolve a tablespoon at a time in a tablespoon of boiling water until the mixture thickens.

Dissolve any of the gums in the same way. Use either gum tragacanth, gum arabic or gum acacia.

The following recipe can be used with any of the above herbs substituted for the gum tragacanth:

water	¾ cup
gum tragacanth	1 teaspoon
ethyl rubbing alcohol (buy best brand)	¼ cup
glycerine	3 drops
perfume (optional)	3 drops

Boil water in double boiler and stir gum tragacanth on the surface of the water. Do not let powder (or herbs) go lumpy. Add the alcohol, glycerine, perfume. Stir again. Stand overnight to thicken.

For a thicker lotion, lessen the water and alcohol. For a thinner lotion, increase alcohol. The thinned version can be used in an atomizer.

Gelatine

Natural gelatine can also be used as a gelling agent for setting hair, or as a hair body builder for limp or thin hair. For a hair thickening effect, use a packet of the dissolved gelatine plus a whole egg and herbal shampoo. Wash hair with mixture. Rinse.

Small amounts of gelatine can also be added to rinse water to increase the heaviness of the hair. Colored gelatines can be used in the following way: lemon for light hair; raspberry, strawberry or cherry for redheads and brunettes. The sugar in the colored gelatines seems to add additional body, in the same way that sugar in the final rinse water adds body (almost like a starch) to fabrics.

Lemon Hair-Setting Lotion

This lemon-water setting lotion takes a long time to dry but has the advantage of holding a set for a long time. It was described to me by a film makeup man. Use either bottled lemon juice or make up your own from fresh strained lemon juice, or boiled, strained lemon juice. Add a teaspoon of eau de cologne to this lemon, and hold in the refrigerator until you use it.

25. TONICS

Hair is a reflection of the whole person, and if your spirits are low or you have been deprived of adequate food or sleep, this will show up in the form of dull, listless and sometimes falling hair. Brushing should be the first order of attack. Make sure you have a natural-bristle brush and spend that old-fashioned 100 strokes a night on *each section* of your hair. You will see results in a short time.

Under various other headings I have discussed the herbs and combinations that will help revitalize the hair. They are rosemary, sage, nettle, chamomile, castor oil and forms of gum camphor, as well as other stimulating herbs that are listed in various other recipes. For dark hair, rosemary and sage are good tonic herbs; chamomile is best for light hair.

To make a hair tonic with herbs, pour a pint of boiling water over 4 tablespoons of your chosen herb. Steep for several hours. Strain. To preserve this lotion, add a few drops of eau de cologne or a dozen drops of gin. Either massage through hair, or use in shampoo or rinse water.

We discovered one of my grandmother's hair-reviving tonics in a book of her poems. It was the kind of recipe family friends frequently requested. Jaborandi is a stimulating herb. Use only *ethyl* rubbing alcohol, or a strong-proof vodka.

jaborandi	1 ounce
nettle	1 ounce
rosemary	1 ounce
ethyl alcohol (or vodka)	6 ounces
castor oil	12 drops
perfume	5 drops
salicylic acid	¼ ounce
distilled water	4 ounces

Soak jaborandi, nettle, rosemary in the alcohol for 3 weeks. Strain into another container. Add castor oil and perfume. Dissolve salicylic acid in distilled water. Add to herbal and oil solution. Use as a nightly massage.

Another hair-reviving herb is gum camphor, USP. Steep 1 ounce of crushed gum camphor and 2 ounces of powdered borax in 2 quarts of boiling water for several hours. Keep refrigerated. Use as a nightly massage on scalp.

26. DANDRUFF

According to prominent skin and hair specialists, dandruff can be caused by faulty diet, stress, hormonal disturbances, infections, injury to the scalp and the increased used of injurious hair preparations, especially those that claim to control dandruff.

Dandruff is simply the sloughing off of matured skin cells through the pores of the scalp. It is only when flaking becomes excessive that it has to be considered a problem. Well-brushed, clean *healthy* hair with the proper balance of acid doesn't have problem dandruff.

There are two forms of dandruff, one oily and one dry. The oily form is found most often among adults and adolescents with an excessively oily skin and scalp. The same adolescents who have acne often have dandruff too. The cause is the same, an excess secretion of male androgen hormones which has activated the internal skin oil, sebum. Surplus sebum is released through the scalp as well as through the pores of the skin. To control this form of dandruff, many dermatologists and nutritionists restrict the food that also stimulates acne. Eat less animal fat, and only use monounsaturated or polyunsaturated vegetable oils on salads. Olive oil is great. *Don't* eat butter or fried foods, nuts, chocolate, shellfish, iodized salt. But do eat a diet high in all kinds of salad greens, and green vegetables and yellow vegetables. Cut down on sugar-loaded foods, and replace them with small amounts of nonfat protein such as fish, chicken, turkey or tofu. Add the supplements vitamins E, B complex and A and 500 mg of magnesium daily to your diet.

Brushing

Vigorous daily brushing is important in ridding the hair of dandruff and increasing circulation of the scalp.

Shampoos

Use herbal or Castile shampoos and avoid all synthetic preparations for dandruff, some of which use too powerful drugs. Many are simply irritants which temporarily remove the dandruff, but most cause the scalp to produce more oil to protect itself. Some hairdressers tell me that the side effects of some of the dandruff remedies on the market are falling hair, excessive oiliness and allergic reaction. Some chemical hair sprays also *cause* flakiness and dandruff.

Vinegar

To overcome most dandruff and scalp itching, massage diluted or undiluted apple cider vinegar onto the scalp. To create an aromatic vinegar, add lavender water (or another aromatic *water*) to the apple cider vinegar.

Oil

Oil is an excellent hair aid. Castor oil strengthens the hair. Use it in a hot pack. Other oils which make up superior hair oil packs are hot olive oil, hot flaxseed oil (from health store, not hardware store). These packs, which are also superb for dry hair problems, can be used twice weekly until the dandruff problem is solved.

After massaging the oil into the hair, bind the area with some plastic to keep the heat in, add a shower cap or two, and allow the oil to seep into the hair for at least half an hour. The treatment can be left on for hours. Shampoo with a nondetergent shampoo in an olive oil, coconut, castile or avocado base.

Nettle

Of all the traditional herbal remedies, nettle is the most admired for hair restoration, and is highly regarded in controlling dandruff. An excellent nettle juice is available in health stores for both internal and external use. You can make an instant infusion with two tablespoons of the natural juice plus a pint of boiling water, or use 4 tablespoons of dried nettle leaves and a pint of boiling water, steep for at least an hour. Strain. To either mixture add ¼ cup apple cider vinegar, and 2 or more tablespoons of eau de cologne. If the hair is also oily, you can increase the eau de cologne. Massage this preparation onto the scalp each night.

Rosemary

The easily obtained kitchen herb rosemary is a favorite hair remedy, and is particularly useful in controlling dandruff. There are various rosemary tonics on the market to revive dull and listless hair. A rosemary tonic helps to maintain waves and curl. A light tonic for gentle massage through the scalp can be made by creating a strong infusion of rosemary leaves. Strain. Add either a tablespoon of eau de cologne or a pinch of borax. You can also combine a strained rosemary infusion and sage leaf infusion to produce a very stimulating hair massage. Any of these preparations can be massaged through the scalp or added in small amounts to hair shampoo or final rinse water.

Other Dandruff Chasers

At the first sign of dandruff, massage the scalp each night with witch hazel extract from the drugstore, or diluted lemon juice, or rose water or willow-bark tea. Optional: add a pinch of borax or a teaspoon of eau de cologne.

27. HAIR GROWTH

The loss of hair through illness or vitamin and mineral deficiencies can often be reversed through diet and actions to prevent further stress. I recently met a young man who *had* reversed his hair loss with scalp massages and exercises, daily rests with his feet higher than his head, a shift of diet to organic, pesticide-free food, and high doses of vitamins. Although he had been bald, with this regimen he was able to grow a fuzz in 3 months. By 8 months he had longer hair in many parts of his head, and was still growing baby-soft hair in others.

Still other examples of a reverse of hair loss after illness are mentioned by Peter Flesch in *Physiology and Biochemistry of the Skin*. He states that researchers have recorded good results from the use of B vitamin pantothenic acid. He describes a German experiment on a hypothyroid child whose "scant hair could not be restored by thyroid medication, even though other symptoms of hypothyroidism were alleviated. Administration of pantothenic acid brought about a dense growth of scalp hair."

Quince is used by the Arabs to increase the growth of the manes and tails of their beautiful horses.

Other useful herbs mentioned in old herbals and family recipe books are mallow roots, maidenhair fern spores, nettles, parsley seed, jaborandi, rosemary, boxwood shavings, nutmeg, willow leaves, cloves, artichokes.

The mallows may be boiled in wine and used as a massage. Maidenhair spores are boiled in wine in strong decoction; add white wine and massage through the hair. The parsley seeds are crushed and applied in powder form to the scalp once a month. Allow to remain overnight and brush out thoroughly.

The nettle infusion, or pure plant juice, can be combed through the hair, using an opposite stroke to natural direction of hair growth. Use daily if you can.

In *The Art of Cookery Made Plain & Easy, by a Lady*, 1760, occurs the following note:

An Approved Method Practiced by Mrs Dukeley,
The Queen's Tyre Woman,
to Preserve Hair and Make it Grow Thick.

Take one quart of white wine, put in one handful of rosemary flowers, half a pound of honey, distill together; then add a quarter of a pint of oil of sweet almonds, shake it very well together, put a little of it into a cup, warm it blood warm, rub it well in your head and comb it dry.

Baron Dupuytren's Hair Growth Pomade

The baron gained world-wide fame for this pomade, which he claimed overcame baldness:

rosemary spirits	2 ounces
nutmeg spirits	½ ounce
ethyl alcohol (or vodka)	12 ounces
boxwood shavings	6 ounces

Obtain rosemary and nutmeg spirits at drugstores or botanical

NUTRITIONAL SUPPORT FOR HAIR PROBLEMS

PROBLEM	NUTRITIONAL TIPS
	In general need vitamin A and E and B complex (with choline) plus balanced minerals, plus GLA oil or unsaturated fatty acids capsules every day
DRY HAIR/SPLIT ENDS	Add oils to diet—mono or polyunsaturated oils in salads, and capsules: GLA oil or unsaturated fatty acid capsules
Dandruff	Possible deficiency of one or all of these vitamins: A, B6, B12, and mineral zinc. Need several months of supplementation to see results
Dull hair	To achieve shiny hair add vitamin A foods and supplements, and vitamin A helpers, choline (B vitamin) and vitamin E (helps with color and brightness of hair). Need GLA oil capsules or capsules unsaturated fatty acids. To make the hair more lustrous and manageable, add high dose of vitamin B complex with significant amount of B3 (niacinamide)
Hair falling out Temporary: many women experience a temporary hair loss about three months after delivering a baby, or discontinuing birth control pills	*Minor hair loss:* eat foods rich in iodine, sulphur, iron, silicon or add general balanced mineral supplement to vitamin supplement. Note: Vitamin A is not water soluble and if there isn't enough need for it, or the body isn't absorbing it, a 25,000 IU dose can act like an overdose and *bring about hair loss.* *Serious Hair Loss:* (alopeciatotalis)—nutritional support is help but not total cure. These nutrients have been successful: vitamin A, large doses of vitamin C (immune help), B6, pantothenic acid (B family vitamin), calcium and zinc
Thinning hair	If hair is starting to thin out check for possible vitamin and mineral deficiencies. There may be a B6, or folic acid (B family) deficiency. Minerals such as iron, iodine, sulphur, silicon can act to prevent hair loss
Slow hair growth	B complex foods and vitamins are involved with hair growth. General approach: high B complex supplement after every meal—B6, B12, PABA, Pantothenic Acid, Inositol specific to growth. Also add zinc and vitamin A to diet
Men: no beard	Add zinc supplements to diet as it may be due to low level of mineral. Check for other vitamin and mineral imbalances

sources. To make boxwood, rosemary or nutmeg spirits, for 10 days submerge the herbs in vodka or ethyl alcohol. Strain off the herbs and discard. Combine all the spirits and apply to the scalp for an exceptionally stimulating daily massage.

Artichoke Lotion

Antoine Millet of Paris told me the French country people use this easy formula against baldness.

Simmer a dozen artichoke leaves in a cup of water for several hours. Strain and apply nightly as massage. Store in labeled jar in refrigerator.

Catnip

Many European Gypsies use a catnip infusion as a hair rinse to increase hair growth, stimulate scalp circulation and sooth scalp irritation.

28. HAIR COLORING

There are many natural methods of restoring gray hair to its earlier color, and of changing one hair color to another. One newer concept is the use of vitamins to overcome possible deficiencies, either from malabsorption or illness.

The vitamins that are highly regarded in relation to restoration of color, the anti-gray vitamins, are PABA (para-aminobenzoic acid), calcium pantothenate, choline and inositol. There have been many successful experiments with these vitamins, but legal restrictions on vouching for such vitamin therapy are so stringent that no reliable vitamin producer will allow himself to be quoted on this subject at this time, although privately they admit they have seen results.

To darken hair, the late Dr. Carlton Fredricks advised using the above vitamins in a strong B complex base and also eating milk, brewer's yeast, whole wheat, whole rye, shellfish such as oysters, clams, shrimps and meats such as liver, sweetbreads, and lean pork and ham. He warned that it will take a while to achieve results. PABA had been used in two experiments by Dr. Benjamin Sieve of Boston on patients who had *gray* hair for 2 to 24 years. In 3 to 8 weeks the 800 gray-haired patients who were given this vitamin showed hair changes. Those who had had light hair before they were gray now had dirty-yellowish hair, and those who had dark hair before they were grey found that their hair changed to a darker, dusty grayish color. While these particular experiments are not conclusive, they indicate that PABA may have an effect on gray hair.

Other nutritionists advise drinking a mixture of 2 tablespoons each of apple cider vinegar, uncooked honey and blackstrap molasses in a glass of water every morning. This drink is reenergizing for the entire system and often helps restore hair to its earlier color.

Plant and Vegetable Hair Coloring

Most of the dyes on the markets today are aniline, which is a coal-tar product. Peter Morell, in *Poisons, Potions and Profits*, says, "Hair dyes probably lead the list as the most dangerous of all widely used cosmetics. Aniline dyes can be very injurious to those who are sensitive to such chemicals, and the damage may be of such varied nature that it would be difficult to trace the dye that causes it."

Our forebears discovered the value of leaves, barks, roots, nuts and flowers as coloring material, and over the centuries various combinations came into use. Dark women in Greece and Rome sometimes dyed their hair golden with a mixture of quince juice and privet, while the raven-haired women of Turkey created a supple, shiny, black effect on their hair with a preparation of gall-nuts, first dried in oil and rubbed in salt and then added to a complicated combination of crushed pomegranate flowers, gum arabic, henna and that uniquely Turkish invention, *rastik-yuki*, which is a combination of iron and copper. Arab women, on the other hand, used just henna for auburn shades or henna and indigo to create a blue-black combination, or for simpler effect an essence made of green oranges steeped in oil for several weeks to conquer gray hair.

Many of the plant and vegetable substances which are useful for dyeing can be added to your herbal shampoo.

Henna Coloring—Brown, Auburn, Black, Red

Henna is a nontoxic dye which is not a primary sensitizer or irritant. It has been used for thousands of years in the Near and Far East. Unfortunately, henna dyeing is a long, tedious process, and it is rather difficult to stabilize the color except with experience. The color lasts several months, however, and with experimentation you can achieve a rich auburn, brown or black or an interesting red. Since henna is slightly astringent, be sure to rub a light covering of safflower or corn oil on your scalp before using it.

Hair must be shampooed before using henna. Wear gloves during the entire application as henna can stain hands and fingernails. (For henna nail-polish application see Chapter VII.)

henna powder	2 cups
warm water	1 cup
pure vinegar	1 teaspoon

optional

goldenseal root (powdered)	½ teaspoon

Stir henna powder and water into thick paste. Add vinegar to help release dye. Add optional goldenseal. Let stand for one hour. Stir the henna, vinegar, golden seal in the top of a double boiler until the water in the bottom pot boils vigorously. Remove from flame and let stand for 1 hour. Heat up again quickly, and with gloved hands massage into hair. Cover hair with a linen towel. For brown hair wait for 3 to 4 hours. For auburn or dark hair color let the color stay in up to 6 hours. Then wash the hair. Keep rinsing *and combing the hair as you rinse*, until the water becomes clear. To counteract drying action, gently massage drops of oil into the scalp.

Other Red hair Dyes

There are several other vegetables that will dye the hair a reddish color. A strong infusion of radish and privet mixed together and washed through the hair will turn it red. Saffron will also give the hair a reddish tint, as will marigold flowers.

Other Black or Brown Hair Dyes

Walnut shells make another harmless dye which progressively adds color to the hair. Before the nuts are ripe, crush the green outer shells in a mortar and cover with water. Add a touch of table salt. Let stand 3 days. Now add 3 cups of boiling water and simmer for 5 hours, always making sure the evaporated water is replaced. (Make a mark on the pot.) Express the dark liquid from the shells by means of a press or by twisting the shells in a cloth. Replace separated liquid in pot again and now reduce to a quarter of its volume. Add a dozen drops of perfume if you wish, and some fixative of alum and a touch of glycerine to soften the hair. Use on shampooed, clean hair. At first it will produce a somewhat yellowish effect, but it will finally give the hair a good deep black color.

Other woods which can be used for dyeing the hair are catechu, logwood, brazilwood, quebracho, sandalwood and some redwood. Make a decoction of 4 tablespoons of any of these woods in a pint of water. Simmer for 20 minutes to ½ hour. Strain and brush through hair again and again. Also rinse through hair. These are progressive dyes. Best results will be seen after several applications.

Culpeper says "hair of the head washed with berries [elderberries] boiled in wine is made black."

Golden Hair Dyes

Many Nothern Italian women have the natural golden-red hair immortalized by the Venetian painter Titian and the Florentine painter Botticelli, particularly in his "Birth of Venus." During the Venetian ascendancy as a sea power, especially during the Renaissance, this exquisite hair color was duplicated with dyes throughout the world. The color was so distinctive that there are many references to it in literature, where it is referred to as *capelli file d'oro* (golden-thread hair). Titian's cousin, Cesare Vicallio, reported that many dark-haired Venetian and other Italian beauties who wished to attain this color, spent "hours under the solana, a special crownless hat with a huge brim which was used to spread their long hair on as they sat on the roofs of their palazzos to dry their hair after it had been dipped in liquid dyes."

I do not know the formula for golden-thread hair, but it was probably henna with some citric acid base.

Chamomile

This white-and-yellow flower lightens mousy or blond hair. You can use it either as a rinse or as a dye. If you just want highlights, infuse a handful of the flowers in a pint of boiling water, steep for a few hours and strain. As with all *special rinses*, arrange to have an extra basin to catch the drippings so that you can keep rinsing your hair until the color is right.

For a rinse, make a strong infusion by adding 1 pint of boiling water to 2 to 4 tablespoons of chamomile flowers. Steep for 20 minutes to 3 hours. Strain, and rinse through hair again and again. For a dye, make a paste of 1 cup of the infusion and ½ cup of kaolin clay. Apply paste to hair for varying periods from 15 minutes for a lightening effect to 60 minutes for a warmer blond tint.

For extra highlights to rinse or dye add quassia chips. First simmer chips to soften them and add to chamomile while steeping to make infusion. Strain.

Rhubarb Root Golden Dye

This is by far the most effective herbal hair lightener that I have experimented with. Even the very first rinse or application results in a heavenly honey-gold look, which becomes softer and deeper gold as it is applied again. If you can sit in the sun after using it, this seems to enhance the color and strengthen the effect of the dye. Rhubarb roots can dye dark blond hair golden, or lighten brown hair to a rich golden color. Use gloves with this dye as it can stain the palms and fingernails, although it washes off quite easily.

rhubarb root	4 tablespoons
water	1½ pints
(or white wine)	

Simmer root in water or wine for 20 minutes. Steep for several hours. Strain twice. Rinse through the hair several times or use as a paste. Paste will dye hair more effectively, especially at the roots. To make the paste, add ½ a cup of kaolin powder to a cup of decoction. (To counteract possible drying action add beaten egg yolk and ½ tesaspoon of cider vinegar and a teaspoon of glycerine to condition the hair). The wine in fact works best, but is quite sticky and must be rinsed off, whereas the water infusion can be left on the hair.

Saffron Dip

Trotula, a famous ancient doctor, left the following recipe. For making the hair golden mix equal parts of elder bark, flowers of broom and saffron, plus the beaten yolk of an egg boiled in water. Skim off the pomade that floats to the surface and use as a hair dye.

Mullein

Mullein are tall, candle-shaped plants with long, fuzzy, green leaves and tiny yellow flowers. The stately mullein stands alone, in meadows and wastelands. Once you recognize this plant, you will see it again and again as you drive along highways and through rural areas. The yellow flowers produce an excellent healing oil for ear infections. The leaves produce a wonderful liquid which will produce a lovely golden hair color. Simmer the leaves, steep, and carefully strain out liquid—you may have to do this with a fine mesh—and rinse through the hair. Mullein oil is available through many botanical sources.

Honey Dye

Another successful old-fashioned and harmless dye is made of honey and gum arabic. But it is quite difficult to make unless you possess either an old-fashioned perfume still or a modern water distiller. It was thought to be nourishing and effective blond dye for the hair.

"Take the best honey, 2 pints, gum arabic 2 ounces. Distill with a gentle fire. The first water which come forth doth whiten the face, the second and the third make the hair yellow."

To Turn Gray Hair Dark

People have always spent a lot of time and money working out "waters" to darken the hair to its original color. Ralph Harry points out that it is unlikely that such historical personages as Marie Antoinette or Sir Thomas More *suddenly* turned gray while in prison. "Hair washes and dyes have been known since the earliest days," writes Harry. "In the case of political and other prisoners, it is more than likely that those incarcerated no longer had access to their favorite dye. Uncharitable, but possibly a much more likely scientific explanation of any such occurrence."

Among the dyes for darkening hair and hiding the gray are infusions of leaves of the wild vine, artichoke, mulberry tree, fig tree, raspberry bush, myrtle; decoctions of roots of the holm oak and caper tree; decoction of barks of the willow, walnut tree and pomegranate; decoction of shells of beans, gall and cypress nuts; green shells of walnuts, ivy berries, cockles; red beet seeds, poppy flowers, alum. Also sage, marjoram, balm, betony, laurel infusions.

The Arabs use the essence of green oranges steeped in oil for several weeks to restore color to graying black hair.

An old recipe says your hair will turn black if, after you have washed it, you dip your comb in oil of tartar and comb it through three times a day while in the sun.

Dried or fresh sage will darken gray hair. It can be added to the shampoo and also used as a rinse. Make a strong infusion of at least 4 tablespoons to a pint of boiling water, and apply the strained and steeped liquid with a sponge or cotton wool to the roots of the hair. A long-lasting sage hair-darkener can be made with a pint of dark sage tea, a pint of bay rum and 1 ounce of glycerine. Bottle and label and apply to roots each night until hair reaches desired color.

Tag alder root, or red alder, produces another dye which will gradually darken the hair brown. You can experiment with the amount needed but can make a weak solution with 1 ounce and a pint of boiling water. Simmer for 20 minutes, steep for several hours, strain and use with sponge or cotton wool on roots of hair. To preserve, use the same proportions of bay rum and glycerine as in the sage recipe.

CHAPTER V

EYES

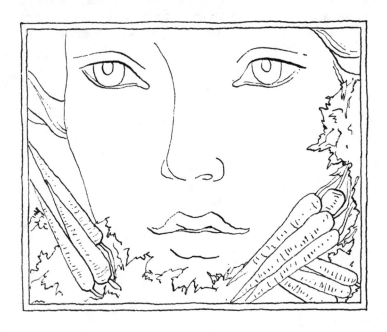

Have you ever noticed how quickly your eyes respond to negative and positive stimuli? How shiny and bright they look when you are happy and relaxed, how dull when tired? How smog and smoky rooms make them bloodshot, and how lack of sleep will cause shadows and puffiness under them? The eyes are intimately connected with the brain and other parts of the body, and immediately reflect unhappiness or malfunctioning—

as with the yellow look from a gall bladder or liver attack, for instance.

Food and the Eyes

Though I am a supporter of many old remedies and herbal aids, it becomes more and more obvious that all these aids must be used in conjunction with cleansing and purifying foods, and foods which will regenerate the cells and revitalize your complexion, your hair and the rest of you.

One of the earliest food–disease connections was the brilliant observation of Egyptian doctors of the affinity between many diseases of the eye, and how eating liver often cured these eye diseases. This worked because liver contains high amounts of vitamin A, a vitamin essential to good eye health. In addition to A, eye health demands adequate intake of vitamins C and B every day, as well as other supplements and trace minerals.

In the past physicians also wrote about the possible connection between eye health and the digestive system. One of my favorite turn-of-the century herbalists, Jethro Kloss in *Back to Eden*, says that eye troubles "are caused mainly from a deranged stomach," and advises readers to eat fruits, fruits juices, cucumbers, carrots, celery and leafy vegetables to cleanse one's system. He says, "Eat foods which will give you a pure bloodstream." Since digestive problems have such an impact on eye health, consider this anticonstipation measure: a glass of pure, *cold* water first thing in the morning. Some people like to also add the cleansing juice of lemon to this drink. Another natural drink with a cleansing effect is a glass of water plus a tablespoon of apple cider vinegar, or a tablespoon of honey added to the apple cider vinegar. This last remarkable combination tends to rebalance the body, and when used on a consistent daily basis, can act to dissolve accumulated crystals. For this reason this drink can help to control, and sometimes overcome, arthritis and some cases of gout.

Several vegetables are very helpful for eyestrain. Carrot is the most important, since it contains a large amount of vitamin A. Others are celery, parsley, chicory, spinach and escarole. I tried these when having trouble with my own eyes, when new glasses and eye exercises were not proving completely successful, and the effect was excellent. Make juices with an extractor, using fresh washed vegetables, preferably those which have not been sprayed with pesticides.

29. SLEEP

A renowned 19th-century beauty wrote that the best recipe for bright eyes is keeping good hours: "Just enough regular and natural sleep is the great kindler of woman's most charming light." Many models have told me that they couldn't function, and their eyes would start looking crepey, if they didn't get between 8 and 10 hours' sleep a night. Most people function well on 7-8 hours sleep. As they get older many people sleep shorter periods at night.

Resting During the Day

Some people are born with an inexhaustible amount of energy. Others need to rest sometime during the day. If you were normally energetic during the day, but have a recent pattern of daytime fatigue, these ideas may help.

Add 15 minutes of relaxing stretching to your early-morning routine.

Do 10-15 minutes of some energized exercise—it could be vigorous walking, or simply dancing to your favorite music.

Recheck your diet to see if it contains enough raw vegetables and fiber.

Lower the fat intake (changing from regular milk to skim, and cutting down on all red meats is a good start).

Add a good all-around B complex supplement and foods and some acidophilus yogurt or capsules.

30. EYE REFRESHERS

Fresh cucumber is inexpensive and readily available. It is a magnificent eye aid, as it tones the membranes while it cools and soothes inflamed eyes. The juice alone, squeezed in and around the closed eye, has a calming effect. Peel and thinly slice two rounds of cucumber. Lie down comfortably. Apply a slice of cucumber to each eye for instant relief and eye pleasure.

Witch Hazel Extract

Witch hazel was one of the many herbal discoveries of American Indian tribes. It was used by the pioneers and it is still available in local drugstores as witch hazel extract. Among its many uses I like it to reduce inflammation on the skin, and puffiness around the eyes. Soak cotton puffs or a clean handkerchief in the extract (use the reliable Dickenson brand) and apply over closed eyelids for almost immediate relief from puffiness, eye fatigue, eyestrain, sunstrain, tears.

Eyebright

My grandmother was never without a jar of strong infusion of the revered old herb eyebright in her icebox, and I follow her example by keeping some at all times in my refrigerator. I use it whenever I can. Father Kunzle, the Swiss master-herbalist, in *Herbs and Weeds* reports that the whole herb is used to strengthen the eyes, and that the "ancients boiled it in wine and drank it at bedtime." Father Kneipp, in *My Water Cure*, also recommends it for washing the eyes.

Recently a friend came to my house after a long tiring day, and while we were dressing for the opera she asked if I had anything for the dark circles under her eyes. I mentally hovered over several remedies, but finally suggested the ice-cold eyebright—and a 15-minute rest. The circles lightened and almost disappeared.

Chamomile, Wormwood and Other Herbs

Chamomile infusion is also a favorite eye aid and is very soothing when used as a compress.

Wormwood infusion is effective for eye inflammation, while a horsetail decoction will bring down swelling of the eyelids.

Jethro Kloss recommends 1 teaspoon of *red raspberry leaves*, 1 teaspoon of *witch hazel leaves* in a cup of boiling water for a wet eye pack. Strain to use. He also recommends fennel tea as a drink and for eye bathing (dilute the tea by a third). Also highly recommended is one of his favorite herbs—*goldenseal* mixed in equal parts of 1 teaspoon each with *boric acid* in a pint of boiling water. Shake, allow to settle and then apply to closed eyelids. Fennel, eyebright and chamomile can also be used together for soothing the eyes, Use ⅛ teaspoon each of dried herbs in 1 cup of boiling water, strain, cool and soak in cotton pads and apply to closed eyelids.

Eat carrots, endives, strawberries, parsely and potatoes to strengthen the eyes.

31. PUFFINESS AND CIRCLES

Dark circles under the eyes can emerge because of illness, insomnia, fatigue or strain. Sometimes such dark circles are nature's way of telling us to get more rest. If the circles emerge and do not go away after a time, they may signify a need to flush the kidneys with water. At physical checkups, those with potential kidney problems are usually advised to flush the body with at least 8 glasses of water each day. A good way to do this is to buy quarts of bottled water in advance. Each morning take out 2 bottles. It often helps to drink several glasses early in the morning. At any rate, when the 2 bottles have emptied you know you have reached the daily required quota of water. To avoid flushing away essential potassium as you do this, make sure you also replace the potassium with either a whole orange, some grapefruit or a banana each day.

Swollen lids sometimes surface during a cold, from an allergy, or after crying. Such spontaneously swollen lids respond to a series of cold packs or cold witch hazel compresses. If the swelling becomes chronic, check this symptom with your physician.

NATURAL DIURETICS

Foods	Asparagus Asparagus tincture 16 drops in a glass of water Watermelon meat Parsley soup
Herbs	Nettle juice Uva Ursi Lady's mantle Beard of corn Couch or quick grass
Bottled waters	Some mineral waters act as minor diuretics

32. CREAM FOR BELOW THE EYES

There is no such thing as a cream to *eliminate* wrinkles, but the following eye cream will clean the area under your eyes—a delicate area prone to dryness—and keep it lubricated and soft. The eyes are very delicate. If you are allergy-prone, first test the cream in a small area.

anhydrous lanolin (solid or liquid)	3 tablespoons
mineral oil	1 tablespoon
egg yolk	1
beeswax	2 tablespoons
safflower oil	2 tablespoons
cold water	1 tablespoon (optional)

The mineral oil is included here because it helps cleanse eye makeup from the eyes. If you prefer, you can use a tablespoon of melted lanolin instead.

Melt the lanolin and mineral oil together in a double boiler until the mixture gels a little. Add beaten egg yolk. In another double boiler melt beeswax and safflower oil. Add the beeswax and the safflower oil to the lanolin, mineral oil and egg yolk. Add water if you wish, as this helps moisturize, though the water sometimes gives the cream a smarting effect. Beat the mixture until frothy. Jar and label.

33. EYE EXERCISES

STRENGTHENING THE EYES WITH EXERCISES

Ceiling-to floor	Lift eyes to the ceiling. Shift to the floor. Repeat 3 times. Gradually increase to 10 times
Right diagonal	Lift your eyes on a right diagonal to the ceiling. Hold. Shift eyes to the opposite corner diagonally to the left. Hold. Rest. Repeat 3 times. Gradually increase to 10 times.
Left diagonal	Lift your eyes on a left diagonal to the ceiling. Hold. Shift eyes to the opposite corner diagonally to the right. Hold. Rest. Repeat 3 times. Gradually increase to 10 times.
Circles/clockwise	Practice first with clockwise half circles on the top area and on the bottom area. As soon as the eye accepts the circle concept, start to slowly make full clockwise circles. Make a circle with both your eyes by shifting them up on the left, round to the right, down again on the right and over to the left. Rest. Repeat 3 times. Gradually increase circling ability until you can make smooth clockwise motions. Circling rate may be increased as you gain muscle control.
Circles/anticlockwise	After accomplishing clockwise motions, try the same motions in counter-clockwise manner.
Finger straight ahead at distance. Use this exercise to relax eyes when you are reading or doing any close work.	Use index finger. Hold it about two feet from your nose. Focus eyes at distance. gradually move the index finger towards the tip of the nose, allowing the eyes to change focus as you do so.

The Cat

The following relaxing exercise can be done at any time, but it is most effective in the early morning when your eyes are rested.

Get down on your stomach and lie with your head to one side, and your arms by your side, palms up. Slowly, as if you were a cat, open your eyes facing the ground and gradually look around to the side and up to the ceiling. Reverse the sequence. Shift your face to the other side and repeat the movement.

Palming the Eyes

Whenever the eyes feel tired you can relax them by rubbing your palms together to cause friction and heat and applying the palms to your eyes.

THREE PALMING METHODS

Rub palms together about six times to cause friction and heat. Do this after eye exercises to relax the eyes.	Place heated palms gently over your eyes with fingers touching the hairline. Let your eyes absorb the full heat and calm darkness of the palms. When the heat evaporates, pull down the fingers so that they stroke the closed eyes several times. Stroke the fingers across the eyes towards the temples.
This method brings blood to eyes and refreshes them.	With elbows supported on a table, cup a warm palm over each eye so that no light can enter. Open an eye into each palm and stare into the blackness for one to two minutes. This method can be combined with the previous one in in which you created palm heat.
Relieves tension of eye muscles and creates additional circulation of eye fluid.	Close both eyes, and press the heels of your hands into your eye sockets until you gradually see "black." This can be done every hour when you are doing close work or reading.

CHAPTER VI

MOUTH AND TEETH

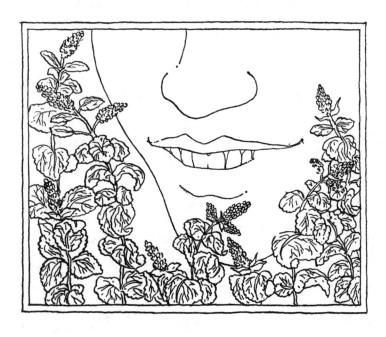

Jack London was first a sailor, then an author and still later a journalist. When he was in a little village in Korea reporting the Russo-Japanese War, the mayor came up to his hotel room to say that the entire populace was gathered in the village square to see him. Naturally London felt quite proud that his writing reputation had preceded him, but when he walked up the special platform they had erected, the mayor only asked him to take out his set of artificial teeth. For half an hour they kept him there taking out his teeth and putting them back again to the enthusiastic applause of the populace.

34. BRUSHING THE TEETH

In bygone days our ancestors used twigs as toothbrushes. My grandmother once showed me how to peel flowering dogwood twigs to cleanse my mouth. She said they had a whitening effect. These days we have a plethora of tooth-cleansing aids, from electric toothbrushes to waxed and unwaxed floss, shaped wooden tooth "picks" to stimulate the gums, threaded "needles" to help floss under bridges, and tiny, tiny brushes to push between and under permanent bridges. All these are vital in keeping up mouth health.

Brushing the teeth not only has a vital cleansing effect, but stimulates hidden energy points on the gums. The newest method of cleansing the teeth is to brush up and down and *across*. It is best to use a soft toothbrush. Even better is a soft, natural-bristle toothbrush.

Coral Sticks

A lovely idea I discovered in an old English herbal is the coral stick. I reprint the recipe in its entirety.

"Make a stiff Paste with tooth powder and a sufficient quantity of mucilage of gum tragacanth. Form with this Paste little cylindrical rolles, the thickness of a large goose quill, and about three inches in length. Dry them in the shade. The method of using these corals, is to rub them against the teeth, and in proportion as they waste, the teeth get cleaner; they serve instead of tooth powders, opiates or prepared roots, but they are brittle and apt to break, and on this account are less convenient than tooth powder that is used with the prepared roots."

Tooth Powders

Lemon peel used occasionally will take the brown stains off the teeth. After using lemon, rinse the mouth thoroughly.

One of the oldest tooth cleansers is common salt with water. Make a light paste and dip the brush into it. Rinse carefully.

Another favorite of mine is the strawberry. Squash a fresh strawberry in the mouth and rub against each tooth. It leaves a delightful clean taste.

Sage was used by the American Indians as a mouth cleanser and is still used today by many Arab people. Use the leaves alone or combine with a touch of honey and charcoal made from bread. As an alternative to sage you can use celandine leaves.

Several roots were once used as the base for home tooth powders. Grind equal parts of bistort root, bayberry root and prepared chalk.

Camphorated chalk has two virtues, being an inert substance and antiseptic. It is therefore useful for dental purposes. Make a paste as follows:

camphor USP	1 teaspoon
sugar	1 lump
crushed almonds	1 tablespoon
distilled water	½ pint

Powder the camphor USP and the sugar. Grind the almonds. Mix together. Add the water and make into a paste.

35. THE MOUTH

Mouthwashes

Sunflower seeds are high in vitamin A, phosphorus, fluorine and calcium, and therefore have a marked effect on the teeth (as well as the eyes) and can help to control bleeding gum condition in a relatively short time.

Rose water can be used as an aromatic gargle and mouthwash. (There is an inexpensive recipe for rose water in Chapter X.)

The following combination of herbs makes a delightful mouthwash. Steep ¼ teaspoon of rosemary, anise and mint leaves in a pint of boiling water. Strain. Pour into labeled jar.

A Spicy Mouthwash

crushed cloves	2 tablespoons
crushed nutmeg	2 tablespoons
ground cinnamon	1 tablespoon
caraway seeds	1 tablespoon
sherry	½ pint
spirits of lavender	10 drops
(or spirits of peppermint)	

Grind all the dry ingredients together in a marble mortar and pour into sherry. Soak for 3 or 4 days and add either the lavender spirits or peppermint spirits. This is a highly concentrated mouthwash. Use only a few drops in a glass of water.

Small amounts of the following herbs can also be used in mouthwashes: mallow flowers, leaves of the bugle, pellitory of the wall, with honey and water.

The best mouthwash of all is probably peppermint infusion. At home we always keep a batch of fresh peppermint "tea" in the refrigerator to use as a mouthwash and a drink. It is very cleansing to the mouth, and as a drink cleanses the entire system. Apple juice, with its natural acids, is also excellent for a home mouthwash.

Many of the old herbals praise lavender water for tooth and gum care. One old recipe book describes it as follows: "Beyond doubt it is of infinite service. This simple and innocent remedy is a certain preservative, the success of which has been confirmed by long experience."

Lavender water not only makes a fine mouthwash, but can be used also in other ways. It is strongly aromatic and can be employed as a cologne, and to scent the bath. When used in a foot-bath, it helps cure body and foot fatigue, and a few drops on the head can alleviate a headache.

Myrrh is a resinous substance that is excellent for the mouth area since it is a mild disinfectant and a local stimulant to the mucous membranes. Myrrh can be melted down and added to any other mouthwash (it acts as a preservative), or purchase a tincture of myrrh at your pharmacist, or herbal shop. Add a few drops to water. Myrrh has been used for centuries to cure or control spongy and ulcerated gums. Use drops of tincture of myrrh alone, or for a stronger effect combine with a pinch of goldenseal powder and apply directly on cold sores, canker sores or gum sores. Honey is also an effective, soothing therapy for tongue and mouth sores. Apply small amounts directly on the sore several times a day.

Vitamin C used daily, especially as part of a multivitamin program, helps to preserve the integrity of the gums.

Balsam for Chapped Lips

Mix 2 tablespoons of clarified honey and a few drops of lavender (or any aromatic) water. Keep in labeled jar and rub on your lips first thing in the morning, or last thing at night before sleep.

Canker Sores

Canker sores sometimes emerge under stressful conditions which can often be controlled with bed rest, careful diet and deliberate relaxation to avoid tension. To control, apply a small amount of combined tincture of myrrh and goldenseal powder directly on the sore. Rinse out with small amounts of diluted tincture of myrrh and the goldenseal powder, then with clear water. Add 100 mg B complex to daily diet.

Herpes Cold Sores

Herpes cold sores usually erupt in the same place. As soon as you are aware of a warning such as puckering, pulling or tingling in that area swing into action by massaging the area with an ice cube. If you catch the prodrome (early warning), you may avert an attack. Herpes also responds to special nutrition and careful stress management.

Breath Sweeteners

It is possible to have a sweet-smelling, tangy and fresh-feeling mouth. Everyone knows that it is absolutely necessary to brush one's teeth, floss between the teeth and rinse the mouth of food debris to keep from having bad breath. What is less known, but just as important for good breath, is the daily need for plenty of pure drinking water, as well as a quantity of high-fiber cereals, grains, fruits and vegetables to increase daily elimination. Chlorophyll supplements and green chlorophyll-rich foods also help keep the breath sweet.

Chorophyll is the green pigment found in plants. Much of the commercial chlorophyll found in breath-sweetening tablets is extracted from nettle. The commercial product is treated with an alkali to change it chemically to a salt (chlorophyllin). You can get the same effect without the alkali, by drinking a combination of nettle juice and pure water, or eating green-rich salads every day. Parsley and watercress are particularly cleansing for the complexion and the system. Tops of turnips and radishes are also high in chlorophyll, and can be added to beets, carrots, celery or apples in a juice extractor.

CHAPTER VII

HANDS

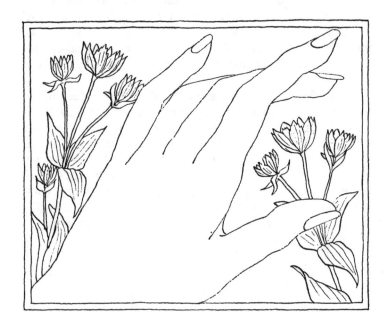

Hands are probably one of the best examples of the double standard. For while most of us respect a man with strong work-hardened hands, and accept the mechanic's or factory worker's stained hands, we expect a woman, no matter what her work, no matter what her age, to have soft, delicate and clean hands at all times. As a city dweller most of the year, a housewife, cook, gardener and full-time writer, I can testify how difficult this is to achieve.

36. HAND PROTECTORS

Replace harsh overalkaline soaps with a glycerine or coconut-oil soap to save the good looks of your hands. If you refuse to wear gloves, it helps to scrape your nails over a bar of soap before doing any dishwashing or mechanical or dirty jobs. Latex gloves for kitchen and other cleaning jobs are an aid in maintaining attractive hands and nails because they prevent broken nails, dirty knuckles, cracked skin and dirt under the nails. Allergists have discovered that a small segment of the population is allergic to latex. This allergy sometimes manifests itself with a runny nose or asthma.

Lemon, Vinegar, Brandy

Lemon halves left over from salad dressings can double as a skin whitener and softener and a nail and cuticle cleaner. It is also a great antidote to fishy hands. Lemon juice also helps restore the acid coating the skin requires. Pat lemon on your elbows to keep them soft and pliable too.

A charming 19th-century toiletry book has the following note: "If the hands are inclined to be rough and to chap, the following wash will remedy the evil: 3 ounces each of lemon juice and white wine vinegar and ½ a pint of brandy."

Ordinarily lemon tends to attract mold after a while, but the brandy and the vinegar preserve it, and each has a special use in hand care. If you prefer, you can use either the lemon or the vinegar alone.

Protective Barrier Cream

If you are doing any particularly hard manual work, make up a vegetable or nut cream protective barrier.

kaolin (or fuller's earth)	1 teaspoon
almond oil	1 teaspoon
egg yolk	1

Mix all three together and rub into hands and under the nails, and around the fingers and wrists. Allow to dry. At conclusion of work, wash off. This is far better for your hands than most chemically prepared protective creams on the market.

37. HAND RESTORERS

Almonds

In an old book, *A Plain Plantain*, I found the following recipe:

Take a pound of Sun Raysons; stone ym; take a pound of Bitter Almonds; blanch ym & beat ym; in stone mortar, with a glass of sack take ye peel of one Lemond, boyle it tender; take a quart of milk, & pint of Ale & make therewith a Possett; take all ye Curd & putt it to ye Almonds; yn putt in ye Rayson: Beat all these till they come to a fine Past, & putt in a pott, and keep it for ye use.

When I discover that I have been neglecting my hands I use a quick version of my grandmother's hand remedy, and it never fails. I take either almond meal moistened with a little milk, or almond oil, and make a paste with a yolk of an egg, a few drops of cider vinegar, and a large spoonful of pure honey. I apply this to my hands and cover them with cotton gloves. Almond oil, by the way, is quite stable and won't go rancid.

Glycerine and Rose Water

Glycerine and rose water is an ancient remedy. The glycerine acts as a moisturizer by obtaining water from the lower skin layer and creating a natural moisture equilibrium.

You will find a glycerine-rose water combination at drugstores, but since this preparation is a bit thick for my taste I often make my own version by using 4 tablespoons of glycerine to every ½ cup of my homemade rose water, which I make by adding a small vial of rose oil to a gallon of distilled water. For a thickened hand-cream version, heat 2 tablespoons of glycerine, 2 tablespoons of corn flour with ½ cup of rose water until it thickens.

Other satisfactory versions of glycerine and rose water are made by adding ¼ teaspoon of either lemon, cider vinegar, or cider vinegar and honey.

A Spanish Pomade

You can use this or any rose water and glycerine as many times as you wish, and certainly it is safer and less taxing than the efforts made in the 1800s by certain Spanish ladies. The 19th-century dancer Lola Montez described their tortures, "Spanish ladies take, if possible, more pains with their hands than with their faces. There is no end of the tricks to which they resort to render them delicate and beautiful. Some of the devices are not only painful, but exceedingly ridiculous. For instance, I have known some of them to sleep every night with their hands held up to the bed posts by pulleys, hoping by that means to render them pale and delicate. Both Spanish and French women—those at least who are very particular to make the most of these charms—are in the habit of sleeping in gloves which are lined or plastered over with a pomade."

Lola Montez described the pomade as consisting of a pound of soap, a gill of salad oil, an ounce of mutton tallow boiled and mixed with a gill of spirits of wine added just before the mixture became cold.

Oatmeal

Oatmeal is another hand cleaner-restorer which can soothe rough or red skin. You can wash or scrub with uncooked or cooked oatmeal cereal, or use the prepared colloidal oatmeal, available in pharmacies under the trade name *Aveeno*. Oatmeal and water were the legendary base for the famed Countess of Jersey's beauty, and she is said to have used a fresh preparation of oatmeal on her hands, face, neck and shoulders each morning to preserve her beauty into a handsome old age.

In many parts of England they still use oatmeal and water plus a few drops of simple tincture of benzoin plus a teaspoon of almond meal as a whitening hand cleaner. For especially chapped hands a 19th-century ladies' manual advised bathing the hands in a mixture of flaxseed (linseed) oil and bitter almond oil, and afterwards rinsing in a water to which simple tincture of benzoin is added.

Cocoa Butter

Cocoa butter is an effective skin softener for the hands. Equal parts of cocoa butter, oil of sweet almonds and white wax (preferably beeswax) can be melted together, stirred until cool and kept in a labeled, dark glass jar.

Cucumber

Cucumber added to the gelling Irish moss (or carragheen) and gum tragacanth, glycerine and a preservative such as alcohol make up a fresh-smelling, long-lasting hand cream.

gum tragacanth	1 teaspoon
Irish moss	1 teaspoon
boric acid	1 teaspoon
borax	1 teaspoon
glycerine	2 ounces
ethyl alcohol (70)	3 ounces
peeled cucumber	

Add a touch of really hot water, enough to mix the gum tragacanth and Irish moss until they dissolve. Add boric acid and borax. When all of these have been completely dissolved add the glycerine and ethyl alcohol and finally the whole cucumber. Blend. Put this into a 16-ounce bottle, add enough hot water to fill the bottle and add a few drops of perfume to your own personal taste.

Hand Care Herbs

Fennel, yarrow, marigold petal, lady's mantle, chamomile and mallow are herbs that can restore chapped or roughened hands.

Boil water, steep and strain and apply a wash of the liquid, or use the mash of any of the herbs in a handkerchief or cloth and apply to the hands.

Do	Do not do
Use gloves for housework	Avoid contact with any harsh chemicals and detergents. Try to keep hands out of water. Nails swell during heavy immersion—there is reaction to the yo-yo effect of immersion and subsequent drying
Scrape nails across bar of soap before washing dishes, or other manual work, or use barrier creams on hands and under nails. Use only a wooden stick to clean under nails	
If using rotary dial phone, use pencil or metal dialer.	
In filing nails, round out. Use emery board, file in *one direction*	Do not file nails in points
Tips: to help avoid drying of nail enamel, add castor oil to *acetone* nail polish. Try non-allergenic enamel. To dry nails faster, plunge them into ice water. For white nails—File, scour with nail brush. Combine white polish and base coat, and paint *under* white of nails.	Avoid using drying nail lacquer or nail polish remover or orange and brown polish (they may make the nail look yellow)
	Don't use press-on nails—they can destroy the nail bed by softening the nail, or separating the nail from skin
Pat oil around cuticles, press with orange stick	*Do not cut cuticles!*
Use nutritional aids to restore strength and general health of nail. Most people need multivitamins. Specific nail problems related to lack of E, C, A, B complex, iron, zinc, calcium.	

38. RECONDITIONING THE NAILS

Have you ever noticed how carefully a doctor looks at your nails when giving you a thorough examination? The nails, like the eyes, hair and skin, indicate your general and specific health. Lack of color, split or soft nails, white spots and cross or longitudinal lines, even dents, are indications and medical history to a trained eye.

39. NAIL AIDS AND POLISH

Cuticle Softener

Combine 2 tablespoons of fresh pineapple juice from raw pineapple, or papaya juice, with 2 tablespoons of egg yolk and ½ teaspoon of cider vinegar. Soak nails for ½ hour. Pineapple and papaya contain an enzyme which softens protein tissue.

Nail Restoration Cream

Combine equal parts of honey, avocado oil and egg yolk plus a pinch of sea salt. Rub into nails. Allow to remain for ½ hour. Rinse off.

Nail Strengtheners

Soak nails for 5 minutes in either warm olive oil, a horsetail infusion, or cider vinegar. Lemon peel rubbed on fingernails strengthens as it cleans and whitens the nails.

Henna Nail Polish

Make a thin paste by adding warm water to henna powder. Apply to nails with a small paintbrush. Allow to dry, preferably in the sun. When thoroughly dry, rinse off in tepid water. This will give you a soft amber pink which will not chip.

CAUTIONARY NAIL PROGRAM

Nutritional Support for Nails

Problem	Use
General health of nail	Calcium tablets, multivitamin
Poor nail growth	May be zinc absorption problem; increase vitamin A
Increase strength of nails	A tablespoon of apple cider vinegar in glass of water before meals, silica (tablet or horsetail tea)
Regeneration of nails	Horsetail tea every night
Peeling nails	Possible vitamin A deficiency
BRITTLE NAILS: avoid immersion in water	Add B complex tablets to diet. Use 500 mg twice a day for 2 months to note change. Also possible calcium deficiency, may need calcium and magnesium. Brittle nails often respond to treatment with lecithin granules or tablets
Thin brittle nails	Check for possible iron deficiency
Brittle nails that peel	B complex, dessicated liver powder in tomato juice. Add silica to diet. 100-200 Vitamin E, vitamin A
Split nails	Add additional vitamin A and vitamin C foods and supplements
White spots on nails	Possible zinc deficiency, also may show low thyroid function
White line across nail	Low in zinc, and may be high in copper
Nails very white, (light-skinned, should be color of skin, dark skin, color of palm)	Need zinc, may indicate too much copper in system

Nutritional Support for Nails

Problem	Use
Hangnails	Need B complex pat vitamin E pricked from capsule on edges of nail until cuticles restored
Soft, damaged nails	Apply vitamin E from capsule on nail for 4 weeks-3 months
Fungus on nail	Daily B complex supplement to build resistance to infection. Apply 2 or more drops vitamin E oil on nail until nail regrows (hand-4-6 months, toe-18 months). Also apply herbal anti fungicides—check tea tree oil and others. At same time *treat internal candida infection! Candida Cleanse (Rainbow)* said to be effective.
Ingrown toenails	First get toenail cut professionally. Afterwards, apply vitamin E to area every day. Good reports on this treatment, but doesn't work for everyone
Flattened nails	Iron deficiency
Concave (spoon-shaped) nails	Iron deficiency
Need to bite nails	May be a systemic need for increased calcium.
Smashed or blackened nails	Massage with vitamin E cream 2-3 times a day
Cloudy white spot on top that travels downwards, means nail is separating, if also yellow-brown color, check for yeast infection in body	Need multivitamins. Use acidophilus, Candida Cleanse, see yeast information in *SuperImmunity For Kids* (Galland and Buchman, E.P. Dutton & Co.)

CHAPTER VIII

FEET

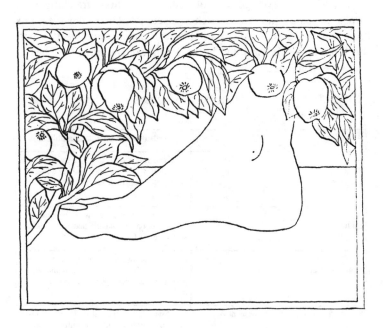

Some time ago the eminent scientist Dr. Harlow Shapley described what he assumed people from another universe might look like *if* they existed. After supplying them with various bodily mechanisms similar to, but not exactly the same as, our own, he conjectured that they would walk not on two, but on *four* legs. Dr. Shapley seemed to think this made more sense. The prevalence of back and foot problems indicates that man was not really made to stand erect on two feet. Learn to pamper your feet with exercises designed to increase circulation and to eliminate accumulated toxins. Cold-water foot baths greatly revive the feet, and strengthen the entire body.

40. EXERCISES

You should never get out of bed without first stretching your limbs and body like a cat. Arch your ankles, bend your toes, flex your entire leg forward, back, sideways and manipulate the toes, heel and ankle forward and back. Whenever you have the chance, massage your feet.

WEAK FEET EXERCISES

Ankles	Flex and rotate as often as possible.
Toes	Flex and rotate each toe by hand. Rise slowly on your toes and go down slowly. Repeat. Pick up marbles with toes.
Entire foot	Walk barefoot on sand, mud or grass. Walk first on the outside and then the inside of each foot.
Legs and feet	Do as much swimming as you can. Walk, kick, lift, fold, knead and massage legs and feet under water in pool or bath.
Herbal foot baths for convalescent or aged	The Swiss master herbalist, Johann Kunzle, suggests foot baths of willow bark.
Detoxification	The German master herbalist, Father Sebastian Kneipp, advises foot and body baths with hay flower. (Extract on market).
	The great British herbalist Culpeper advises foot baths with bed straw.

Draining Away Fatigue

Getting off your feet after an extremely hard day is a good idea, and it helps if you don't merely lie down, but attempt to drain away the accumulated toxins by lying with your feet higher than your head, and gently massaging the legs, one at a time, from the foot to the knee. This helps the circulation and practically pushes the toxins out of your legs. For a 10-minute relaxing exercise, see page 103.

41. HERBS AND BATHS AGAINST FATIGUE

Elderberry

My grandmother wore finely crushed elderberry leaves in her shoes when she felt tired or wished to prevent fatigue. She reduced the leaves to a fine powder in her mortar and usually added a small amount of fuller's earth, to make it into a kind of talcum powder.

Fern

Father Kunzle writes that "people who take long walks will lose every tiredness if they stuff fern leaves in their shoes and fill their pockets with it." Ferns can be found in profusion by the wayside, and also in every florist's shop.

Hot-Cold Foot Bath

Shocking the feet with alternate hot, cold, hot, cold foot baths (ending with cold) will often help eliminate foot fatigue.

Hay Flower Foot Bath

Father Kneipp describes hay flower foot baths as being extremely efficacious for all ailments of the feet, including corns, ingrowing toenails, walking blisters, sweating feet, problem feet of all kinds. He recommends using 5 handfuls of the hay flowers, with stalks, leaves, blossoms, seed, even the hay itself, to a quart of boiling water, and soaking your feet in the tepid mixture. He also mentions oat straw foot baths for corns and other growths. There is a reliable hay flower extract (Biokosma) on the market. Hay flower is also a potent detoxifier for the entire body.

Lavender

A few drops of lavender oil in a tepid foot bath will relieve fatigue immediately.

Lemon or Cider Vinegar Bath or Rub

Lemon juice softens and relieves tired feet. A foot bath in cider vinegar restores vigor to your feet, eliminates itchiness and controls athlete's foot.

Tea Tree Oil

This Australian oil, first used by the Austrialian Aborigines is effective in controlling a number of fungal infections. Rub the oil on affected part.

42. FOOT AND LEG PROBLEMS

Corns and Calluses

Corns and calluses are caused by the way we walk and by friction on the foot. You are therefore better off walking barefoot or with a minimum sandal whenever possible. However, since most of us cannot do this, massaging with olive, castor oil or lanolin, or any favorite face cream, will soften the dead tissue.

Rather than the hay flower baths favored by Father Kneipp, for corns or calluses some herbalists prefer yarrow and salt foot baths followed by a massage with lemon peel oil. You can make this oil by turning half a lemon inside out and steeping your favorite oil in the lemon half overnight.

Another old herbal source mentions that "the juice of houseleek takes away corns from the toe and feet if they be bathed therewith every day, and at night emplastered as it were with the skin of the same houseleek." Houseleek has very healing powers for the complexion, too.

All the root bulbs have drawing power, and garlic or onion tied to corns can ease the pain. Many ancient herbal books mention roasted clove of garlic or onion used several nights in a row as a cure for corns.

Rubbing a pumice stone over calluses softened by bathing will keep calluses small and eventually eliminate them.

Leg Cramps

Father Kunzle suggests a foot bath of boiled water and wood mosses, the kind which can be found along the path in damp woods. Other herbalists recommend cranberry bark, or cramp bark, as it is sometimes called, for quick relief from leg cramps. The herbalists Wood and Ruddock say that people with leg cramps should drink cranberry bark tea night and morning for at least 14 days and "their troubles will seldom return."

Many dancers I know find that large doses of vitamin C and calcium tablets will control and eventually eliminate their leg cramps. Calcium tablets and/or vitamin E capsules are also helpful in stopping the leg cramps associated with menstruation and menopause.

Varicose Veins

Father Kneipp suggests that people with varicose veins should never take baths over 88° F., or foot baths beyond the ankle area. For this complaint, you should always consult your doctor.

Fallen Arches

Fallen arches can be extremely painful and often prevent people from leading an active life. Lucas describes how a liniment of 1 ounce of powdered wormwood, steeped for a week in a pint of rum and then strained and bottled, was rubbed nightly on painful fallen arches and helped one invalid patient return to his work within three weeks. Wormwood is an aromatic herb esteemed by the Greeks as an aid to digestion and appetite, and as an expeller of worms (hence the name). It has a fine reputation as a poultice for all kinds of swelling, sprains and rheumatism.

Homeopathic arnica liniment or ointment can often relieve foot-aches and pain. Use only on unbroken skin.

Itching Feet

Lemon juice and cider vinegar have been mentioned before for itching skin. Either juice can be applied diluted or directly on the skin, or by soaking in a foot bath. Onion juice is an old favorite home remedy and has long been used to relieve itching between the toes. Depending on the severity of the case it can be helpful with athlete's foot problems. The infusion of red clover blossoms, or a wet mash placed in a clean cloth, are other highly regarded remedies for itching of the feet.

Swollen Feet

Father Kunzle has these reassuring words for those whose feet swell in summer. "Do not be frightened, because it is not danger-ous, even though painful. The swelling will soon disappear if you tie crushed red robin [wild geranium] over the ailing spots. At the same time drink tea plentifully made of lady's mantle, or mallow, or of the leaves and blossoms of the bindweed."

The leaves of the house geranium are effective too. Compresses and wrappings with witch hazel extract quickly reduce normal swelling. If the swelling is from retained fluids, use such natural diuretics as parsley tea, uva ursi, watermelon meal, asparagus tinc-ture. Walking in cold water strengthens the feet and other parts of the body.

Foot Powder

If you use a natural powder after the bath you will have less friction when you put on your shoes. The following powder is particularly effective in hot weather:

talcum powder	½ cup
powdered boric acid	2 tablespoons
cornstarch	½ cup
peppermint extract	½ teaspoon
rubbing alcohol	1 teaspoon

Mix the ingredients together into lidded labeled jar.

Perspiration of the Feet

Master herbalist Father Kunzle writes that foot perspiration is "the healthiest illness in existence. It ought never to be quite suppressed because severe and incurable diseases will follow, and will last until the feet perspire again." Father Kunzle advised that this problem be approached by checking on the kidneys. He recommends these herbal diuretics: lady's mantle, Indian corn beard, couch or quick grass for kidney cleansing.

Cold Feet

A tiny bit of cayenne pepper in your shoes or socks will bring you an immediate sense of warmth. To make up in advance as an outdoor talcum powder, add some inert substance such as fuller's earth or talcum powder.

CHAPTER IX

SLEEP

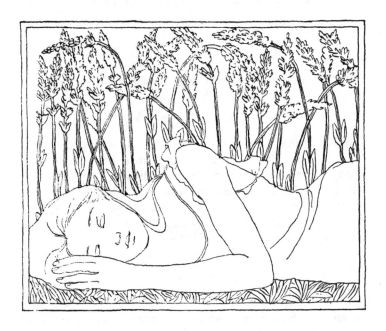

"I often think this insomnia business is about 90 per cent non-sense," said Stephen Leacock. "When I was a young man living in a boarding house in Toronto, my brother George came to visit me, and since there was no spare room, we had to share my bed. In the morning, after daylight, I said to George, "Did you get much sleep?" "Not a damn minute," said he. "Neither did I," I rejoined. "I could hear every sound all night." Then we put our heads up from the bedclothes and saw that the bed was covered with plaster. The ceiling had fallen on us in the night, but we hadn't noticed it. We had 'insomnia.' ''

Leacock was one of the many people who only think they don't sleep; but for people who actually toss and turn the whole night through, there are true physical manifestations. The skin on the face feels saggy and heavy, and lacks tones. Their eyes are bleary and baggy, and their entire body feels dull. On the other hand, a good night's sleep produces a feeling of well-being, freshness and physical energy.

Many people have excellent sleeping habits and only stay awake on the rare occasions when they have something profoundly worrying on their mind, or have eaten too late or over-eaten. Anxiety, cold feet, poor breathing habits and bad circulation are specific causes of sleeplessness. I number quite a few insomniacs among my closest friends, and if they have a single common denominator it is that they are all clever and creative people who cannot, or will not, let their minds stop working. They all say they hate not sleeping, but they won't give up the pleasures of staying up late into the night talking, reading or thinking. Basically they are night people, and they actually wake up physically and psychologically later in the day than other people. I suppose none of them would go along with the adage that ''one hour's sleep before midnight is worth three after.''

Everyone experiences sleepless nights when they go over the day's events, sometimes in a hopeless litany that will not stop. Those who have such ''merry-go-round'' thoughts—thoughts repeated again and again—can often find instant relief in a simple remedy, 4 drops of white chestnut, a Bach Flower remedy. The 38 different flower remedies are available in most health stores.

43. PHYSICAL AND MENTAL RELAXERS

Before going to bed, do some stretches, and take a sitz bath, or a cold water splash to your ankles. If you prefer a long warm bath, try this early 19th-century hydrotherapy strategy—don't towel dry, but instead wrap yourself in a large bath sheet and *pop right into bed under covers.* In a few minutes you'll feel toasty and relaxed. It also helps to breathe deeply. Such deep breaths or deep yawns help to make you feel calm and languid and offset tense thoughts. Breathe deeply 2 to 4 times, and then hold your breath as long as you can. Wait a beat or two and repeat the breathing procedure. Then, as your body and mind begin to feel drowsy, add a touch of autosuggestion. Lie down on your back; slowly and precisely concentrate on your feet, and say to yourself, "My feet are heavy, they feel heavy." Slowly think of each part of your body in the same way. Your legs are heavy, your thighs are heavy, your stomach, your chest, your arms are heavy, heavy, heavy. You feel as if you are floating on water, but now your body is too heavy for you even to lift your arms, your fingers, your wrists. Then mentally make your neck heavy—and then your lips, your nose, your eyes, your head. If you have thoroughly concentrated (and learning this intense concentration sometimes takes a little time), you can fall asleep immediately. But if you find that you are even slightly awake, lie in a comfortable position, preferably with your entire body serenely relaxed, and lift your right foot. Tense it and relax it suddenly. Do the same with your left foot. Lift your right hand. Clench it. Drop it suddenly. Do the same with your left hand. Now tighten your face in a grimace—make an ugly face. Relax it. Give in to the heaviness of your body, if necessary making each part of your body heavy again.

If you are still resisting—and it *is* a matter of resisting—try mentally tracing the number 3—*slowly*. Do this as slowly as you can 3 times, and you should be fast asleep in a short time.

Relaxing Baths

Since relaxed sleep is one of the keys to good health and good looks, all the great herbalist-healers are preoccupied with sleeping aids. Father Kneipp tells of his successful water cures.

Take a cold, 1-second to 3-minute foot bath with water up to the calves. According to Father Kneipp, this will "cure fatigue and produce sound and wholesome sleep."

Another suggested bath is the cold 3-to-5-minute semi-bath, either kneeling in the water so that the thighs are covered, or sitting in cold water which reaches to the pit of the stomach. Father Kneipp claims that these semi-baths are valuable and useful in that they have a great effect on the digestion and intestines. "It serves to regulate circulation, expel unhealthy gases, and make the body impervious to catching colds." These two baths will not only help you to fall asleep, but can be taken to advantage after a bad night's rest.

44. AIDS TO SLEEP

Foods

Calcium and vitamin D are nature's most readily available nightcaps. Warm a glass of whole or skim milk, add a tablespoon of honey and you have an old-fashioned sleeping potion. The calcium tranquilizes and the honey helps the body to retain fluids, thus keeping the kidneys from alerting you during the night. Honey can be used in any herbal tea. Nutritionists also suggest taking 2 tablets of calcium. I like calcium with magnesium.

Suggested *daily* dosages are 1000 mg each of calcium citrate (or gluconate), and magnesium citrate (or gluconate). Also it helps to eat high-carbohydrate foods—these help you to sleep. Before bedtime you might try a baked potato or a slice of bread.

Herbs

The most effective herb sleep-producer in my view is *valerian*, from the Latin *valere*, "to be in health"; it was known to the Greeks as a nerve calmer. To my knowledge, there are no bad aftereffects from the use of this herb, although some people may be sensitive to it. In England it was prescribed to relieve strain brought on by the air raids in the Second World War. Even single doses proved helpful, as it quiets the nervous system and the brain. Unfortunately the dried herb has a bad smell. Use it in coated capsules from herbal pharmacies alone or with other sleep-producing herbs, in capsule or tea form.

Most of the following herbs can be used as nightcap teas. Add

1 teaspoon to a glass of boiling water, steep and strain. Add honey particularly if getting up frequently to pass water. Most tea herbs can be extracted with 15 minutes of steeping; if the time is longer, it will be noted.

Peppermint tea is a delicate and aromatic bedtime drink, and can also be used, as can chamomile, or lime flowers (linden) for babies' sleep and teething problems. Chamomile tea is a traditional tranquilizer and linden or lime (known by its Latin name as *Tilia*) is another effective soothing tea. Even today French mothers give *Tilia* to a crying child, especially at bedtime. Honey from lime flowers is highly regarded for its flavor, and is used in many medicines and liqueurs. Prolonged bathing in lime flower infusion is a folk remedy to calm hysteria. Make sure that you have a reliable supplier for lime-flower tea, as flowers that are too old can produce symptoms of narcotic intoxication. For an old, effective teething remedy combine a tablespoon each of peppermint, skullcap and pennyroyal in a pint of boiling water. Steep for 30 minutes, strain and use warm, with honey for sweetening, 1 teaspoon at a time.

Aromatic woodruff can greatly improve, and even prolong, one's sleep. To make the tea, use only hot, not boiling, water. According to the English herbalist Gerard, pouring woodruff into wine will "make men merry."

A hot mull which will put you to sleep is warm wine plus a few cloves, a stick of cinnamon and a touch of woodruff. Another sleep-producing drink is a toddy with warmed rum, and 6 cloves, 6 coriander seeds, 1 stick of cinnamon, a tablespoon of honey, the yolks of 2 eggs, juice of ½ lemon and a touch of woodruff.

Wild lettuce is narcotic, and all lettuce possesses some of this narcotic juice—not enough to make you drugged, of course. But the ancients held lettuce in high esteem for its cooling and refreshing qualities. In fact the Emperor Augustus attributed his recovery from a dangerous illness to lettuce, and built an altar and erected a statue in its honor. Eau de laitue is water distilled from lettuce, and is used in France as a mild sedative in doses of 2 to 4 ounces. Certainly if you have an urge to eat something before you go to bed, try slowly chewing lettuce leaves, although the teas I have mentioned, plus honey, would be more effective.

Sage is yet another favorite sleep-producer, and a cup of sage tea plus honey will bring on a sense of calm. We always had several "sleep jars" in the house when I was a child, and one jar always contained a teaspoon of sage and rosemary to every 2 tablespoons of peppermint. Use 1 teaspoon of the combined herbs for your steeped, strained tea before going to sleep.

The early American settlers used both *red bergamot tea* and *pennyroyal tea* for relaxed sleep. Lemon balm does double duty in relaxing and stimulation. It doesn't put you to sleep but rather removes any spasms and tensions which prevent sleep; and it can also be used as an early-morning tea to overcome a feeling of tiredness.

Father Kunzle has two suggestions for harmless sleeping potions. He recommends 4 parts of goldenrod to 1 part juniper, or a calming tea of lady's mantle and cowslips combined. Cowslips (*Primula veris*) have been used for centuries in England for nightly tea. Use flowers or root—preferably flowers.

The American herbalist Jethro Kloss advises a warm bath and hot tea for immediate sleep, and he suggests any of the following herbs steeped in a cup of boiling water for 20 minutes: lady's slipper, valerian, catnip, skullcap or hops, especially hops. He says that these herbs will not only induce sleep but will tone up the stomach and nerves, and never leave any bad aftereffect. If none of these herbs is available, hot lemonade, or hot grapefruit juice, either with or without honey, are excellent substitutes.

The Germans use ground anise with honey in warm milk as their bedtime drink, and the Dutch use another version, a tablet of aniseed in a glass of hot milk. Many Indians, I am told, use nutmeg oil on the forehead to induce sleep. The volatile *oil* does contain an intoxicant principle, but even grated nutmeg with lemon and boiling water can sometimes be used as a nightcap.

Many botanical sources and herb pharmacies have their own combinations for sleep. They are frequently made up in the form of capsules.

For sleep aids, Dr. D. C. Jarvis, author of *Folk Medicine*, prefers apple, grape and cranberry juice to citrus juices. Since a great deal of nightly and other unease is due to an overalkaline reaction to the blood, these juices will undoubtedly help. Dr. Jarvis also suggests a daily drink of 2 teaspoons of cider vinegar in a glass of water before breakfast each morning. If you find this difficult to take, try a tablespoon of the cider vinegar and a tablespoon of honey (preferably uncooked honey) to a glass of water, which reconstitutes to a rather apple-juice taste. It is marvellous for getting the body started in the morning, and is an effective cure for constipation—another problem which can affect sleep.

45. HERB PILLOWS

Did your great-grandmother have a sleep pillow—a tiny, slender herb cushion covered with muslin and patterned fabric? These pillows are particularly good for invalids, babies and anyone in need of extra help in sleeping. They are a lovely present for anyone bedridden. The gentle aroma emanating from the pillows soothes the nerves, and helps overcome a sickroom smell.

My favorite of all is lavender, or lavender with crushed rosebuds, or equal parts of sage, peppermint and lemon balm with or without lavender. To help retain the aroma add some powdered orrisroot or a drop of simple or compound tincture of benzoin, as you crush the herbs in the mortar. You can also add a pinch of any of the following: rosemary, lemon verbena (a heavenly clean smell), angelica, tarragon, woodruff, marjoram, dill, thyme, hops.

You can make an entire pillow of hops, or of woodruff, or any of the herbs mentioned before as sleep-helping herb teas. Crush the dried leaves a bit, add a fixative such as orrisroot powder or tincture of benzoin, enclose in a cotton or linen handkerchief and add a washable "pillowcase" covering of a patterned fabric. These should be quite flat and slender to be comfortable. In order not to lose them every time you change your pillowcase, attach with a safety pin to the pillow ticking.

SLEEP TIPS FOR THE SLEEP DEPRIVED

ASK YOURSELF	TO DO	NOT TO DO
SLEEP Am I getting the sleep I need? Do I have many interruptions during the night which make me sleepy the next day?	If you are operating on a sleep deficit you must change your Approach to sleep	Don't ignore persistent sleepy feelings—they are a warning that you need more sleep
CAFFEINE Do I use caffeine during the day to keep awake?	Instead of coffee use herbal teas and vegetable juices such as carrot, beets and celery—these are energizing and cleansing	**NEVER** use caffeine for artificial stimulation. Caffeine and other stimulants actually make you more tired the next day. Caffeine prevents nighttime *REM dreaming* which in turn effects memory, and concentration and in cumulative effect can make one testy, anxious or depressed
NAP If I have insomnia or can't sleep on an occasional basis will taking a nap make my insomnia better or worse?	Catching a **brief 10-15 minute nap** once or twice a day restores vitality, overcomes sleep deficits, and *does help one sleep better at night* If you have to be out especially late one night, **plan** a nap late in the day, or just before you go out	**Never** nap for longer than 10-15 minutes. Long naps put you into a deep sleep which prevents sleep later in the night
Waking up during the night Do I have intermittent insomnia?	If you toss for more than 20 minutes do not stay in bed, instead 1. Turn on light, take pad and jot down anything you are anxious about. Look over the list and pick **one** main worry and write it down in the form of a question (how can I solve . . . ?) or 2. Take a long, warm bath,	

ASK YOURSELF	TO DO	NOT TO DO
	Wrap yourself in a bath sheet and pop back into bed under covers 3. Breathe deeply up to 4 times and hold breath for one count. Repeat or 4. Go to another part of the house, read for a few minutes and then go back to bed	DON'T STAY IN BED IF YOU CAN'T SLEEP
WEEKENDS Do I change my sleep routine during the weekend? Do I go to bed later and get up later in the morning on weekends? How does this hinder or help my weekday insomnia?	Routine is important for insomniacs. GO TO SLEEP AT THE SAME TIME EVERY DAY OF THE WEEK, AND GET UP AT THE SAME TIME IN THE MORNING. Also, insomniacs should create a *personal repetitive* sleep pattern before going to bed every night, e.g., take warm bath, plump out pillows, do certain gentle stretches, breath deeply, etc.	Don't vary the nighttime sleep time or wakeup time, as this affects the body rhythm and contributes to daytime sleepiness
HABITS How else can I adjust my sleep habits?	To avoid daytime sleepiness and get on better routine, start off by going to bed 10-15 minutes earlier every night; continue new pattern for 6-8 weeks	
EXERCISE Does exercise help or hinder good sleep?	Exercise encourages sleep, but to promote sleep it must be done only between noon and 6 PM	NEVER exercise just before going to bed. Don't exercise for 3 hours prior to bedtime, as exercise produces energy and animation and may prevent sleep

CHAPTER X

PERFUMES

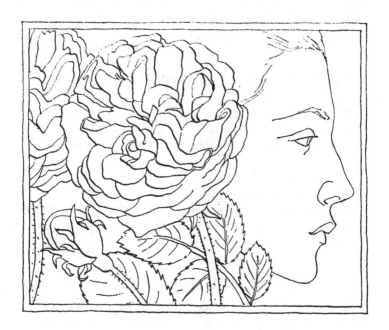

The very best perfumes are blends of several dozen ingredients. These famous perfumes are very expensive, for it takes thousands of flowers to make the best perfume essences. Modern scientific methods are so effective that any woman today can possess scents and perfumes unattainable by the greatest kings and queens of history.

However, it is still possible to obtain or make delightful spicy or floral scents without spending too much money. One way is to buy oils to use as perfume bases or on their own; another is to create your own herbal scents. Most perfumes and colognes require distilling, and whereas many homes possessed stills in the past, they are now frowned upon by the Bureau of Alcohol, Tobacco and Firearms (since whiskey needs distilling). I have therefore concentrated on some old spicy scents that *don't* require distilling—details for potpourri recipes, aromatic waters which have several uses, and scent balls which can be used in cupboards and drawers or be shaped into jewelry.

46. MAKING PERFUMES AND FLORAL WATERS

It is great fun mixing and devising a cologne or perfume for yourself. Buy an aromatic oil in a scent you think you will like at your local health store or from mail order botanical sources.

Floral Waters

Every woman, and many men, of the past used the summery, cool, light scents derived from the orange, and from the flowers of lavender and rose.

Rose and Orange Water

It is impossible to make rose water from scratch without distilling, but nevertheless my favorite rose water is one I make myself, and requires only the mixing together of a gallon of distilled water and 1 ounce of essence of roses. This costs so little that I am quite liberal in my use of such rose water in my bath, or when I want to make an aromatic vinegar, or for various creams, lotions and even shampoos.

Mix the water and essence and let it age for a week or more. The longer the better. You can purchase rose (and other flower) essence from botanical and pharmaceutical sources.

Orange water is made in the same way as rose water.

Lavender Water

In addition to being a complexion water and an old remedy for headaches and fevers, lavender water is a revered scent. It can be eaten on a lump of sugar to allay nervousness or depression. The very best commercial lavender water on the market is Hopkinson's, developed over 250 years ago.

Here are three recipes for lavender water that you can make yourself.

Fragrant Lavender Water

The following is a quick way to give a lavender aroma to water; but it eventually goes bad because of the sugar, so don't make too much of it. Put a lump of sugar and 3 drops of oil of lavender into a pint of clear distilled water, and shake. Use a glass with a narrow neck. After a week or two the water should be usable.

Lavender Tonic

This tonic can be used for the face and for headaches, fevers, nervousness and depression. Grind together in a marble mortar the following ingredients:

dried lavender flowers	2 tablespoons
cinnamon	2 tablespoons
ethyl alcohol or vodka	1 pint

optional

sweet cicely leaves or another aromatic flower	1 tablespoon

Steep for 2 weeks in alcohol. Strain and use.

American Lavender Water

benzoic acid	a few drops
oil of patchouli	½ teaspoon
oil of lavender flowers	½ ounce
oil of cloves	15 drops
oil of wintergreen	15 drops
oil of bay leaves	a few drops
oil of ylang-ylang	5 drops
orange flower water	1 ounce
best grade of ethyl alcohol	

Dissolve the benzoic acid and the oils in the alcohol. Add the orange flower water: shake together well and let stand for 5 days. Filter through a cloth. Label the bottle. Let it stand and age for a few weeks.

47. OLD SCENTS

A Powdered Flower Perfume Base

This can be used as a base for other perfumes, or as a base for talcum powder mixed with corn flour, or alone.

Pound oak moss (lichen) and soak it in distilled or spring water for 5 days. Press out all the liquid. Moisten once again with a combination of rose water and orange water. Keep on soaking the moss until it has fully absorbed the aroma of the roses and the oranges. Press out the liquid. Pulverize the moss and add to any potpourri, perfume or scent ball, or talcum.

An Ancient Spice "Perfume"

Actually this isn't a perfume, but they called it that several centuries ago. It has a very spicy smell which many men like:

rose water	2 cups
bruised cloves	½ ounce
bay leaves	2-3
wine vinegar	2 cups

Combine rose water, cloves, chopped bay leaves and vinegar, and boil. As it reduces, add plain water to bring it to original amount. Put aside in a labeled jar for several weeks or more.

Walnut Leaves and Rose Water

Young fresh walnut leaves and rose water were considered an ideal combination for a man's scent several centuries ago. Heat ½ cup rose water and pour over 2 tablespoons walnut leaves. Steep for 3 hours.

48. POTPOURRI, SCENT BALLS AND PASTILLES

Potpourri is a blending of several dried aromatic flowers or herbs. It can be used to scent a room, drawers or a cupboard, either in a bowl or sewn into sachet bags. You can also scent your writing paper with your favourite potpourri.

General Recipe for Potpourri

There are almost as many recipes for potpourri as there are people who have made them. They depend to a great extent on the fresh or dried flowers you have on hand, and several elementary steps.

In general, rose leaves or lavender leaves should predominate, but don't let tradition confine you. This mixture of scented flowers, aromatic oils and fixative resins and seeds should depend on your personal preference.

If you are a gardener, gather your flowers after the dew has disappeared, and dry the flowers and leaves in the sun until evening.

The key to long life for a potpourri is in the mixture of bay salt and powdered orris root (which is a fine fixative for aromas). Use twice as much bay salt as orris.

Prepare the potpourri in layers: one layer of rosebuds, a layer of orris and bay salt, other layers of flowers, leaves and seeds, rose again, salt and orris again and so on until you come to the top of your jar. Close the lid and put the jar aside in a cupboard for about a month. Then gently mix the ingredients with a wooden spoon and—using either rose or other aromatic oil, or rose water— pour over enough to moisten all the layers completely.

Potpourri Suggestions

Your potpourri does not have to include all these items. Use this list as a guide for developing your own potpourri recipes. When in doubt as to combinations, use rosebuds, small amounts of cloves, nutmeg and cinnamon, and fixatives like gum benzoin, tonquin beans, and some sandalwood, and orrisroot and bay salt as in the general recipe.

For experimental purposes use some or all of the following to *predominate*:

Roses of all colors and shapes, orange blossoms, lavender flowers, lemon blossoms, lilies of the valley, pinks, lilacs, violets, narcissi, heliotrope, jonquils, sweet myrtle leaves, red carnations, jasmine, red bergamot (bee balm), costmary, leaves and flowers of meadowsweet (the favourite room-scenting herb of Queen Elizabeth I), rosemary, woodruff leaves, mint.

Smaller amounts of any of the following: bruised cloves, cinnamon, nutmeg (use two), thyme, sweet marjoram, sage and bay leaves.

Still smaller amounts of the following: yellow sandalwood, calamus root, cassia buds, gum benzoin, storax, tonquin beans.

Scent Balls and Scent Pastilles

Scent balls or scent pastilles are dried aromatic flowers and herbs melted together with a gum resin to harden the mixture. Gums are also fixatives for aromas and will therefore help the aroma to last. They can be made in any size from small-bead size to large-ball size or disks of any size. These will harden so that they can be turned and polished on a lathe and will retain their scent for a very, very long time. If you want to make beads, pierce them with a needle while still quite soft. These scent balls can be used to scent handbags, drawers or cupboards, or in larger sizes can be sculpted into jewelry or belt buckles.

Scent Balls

To make a scent ball, use any group of potpourri ingredients (or use the recipe which follows) and pound them in a marble mortar together with some *gum tragacanth* (the ribbon variety is preferred) and rose water. The gum must be moistened a little with rose water for the whole potpourri to become sticky and doughlike. You can now form this "dough" into any shape you like.

Scent Pastille

powdered orris root	3 ounces
cassia	1 ounce
lavender flowers	1 ounce
cloves	1 ounce
rhodium wood	½ ounce
vanilla	1 teaspoon
tincture of benzoin	6 drops
attar of roses	a pinch, or 6 drops
oil of verbena	15-20 drops
mucilage of gum tragacanth	enough to mix

I have made many variations of these scent balls with odds and ends of different flowers, seeds, gums and leaves, and they have all been successful. Be sure to let them dry in the air. Don't enclose them in plastic, as plastic covering keeps them soft and eventually allows a slight mold to form.

Queen Elizabeth's Perfume

I have included this here as it lends itself particularly to use as a scent ball. It was discovered in an undated manuscript which said, "This perfume is very sweet and good for the time." It *doesn't* endure as a perfume, but with the addition of gum tragacanth (as in the directions above for scent balls) it will last for many years. Like the scent ball, it can also be made into any shape you like.

sugar	2 lumps
rose water	8 tablespoons
sweet marjoram	½ ounce
gum benzoin	2 pieces
(or tincture of benzoin	1 teaspoon)

In a double boiler, crush sugar in rose water and heat. Bring to boil. Add marjoram and crushed benzoin or use tincture of benzoin. Melt and blend the ingredients together. As soon as you can comfortably handle the materials, form into desired shapes.

CHAPTER XI

COLLECTING AND DRYING HERBS

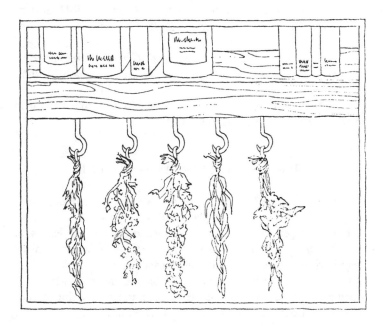

If you live in the country, you will certainly want to investigate the many weeds, wild flowers, roots and barks that you can discover either in your own garden, or by the roadside, or in wastelands or meadows. Before you use these herbs, though, on your body or hair, check whether there has been any spraying in that area. Remember also that by digging up a root you are destroying a wild plant—it may be better to get commercially grown roots from a herbal supplier.

Elizabeth Hall, the late senior librarian of the Horticultural Society of New York, suggests the following four books as basic references in learning about herbs and weeds:

Herbs: Their Culture and Uses, Rosetta Clarkson. Macmillan.

Weeds, Dorothy Charles Hogner. Thomas Y. Crowell.

Weeds of Lawn and Garden, John M. Fogg, Jr. S-H Service Agency, Riverside, New Jersey 08075.

Wildflowers of North Eastern and North Central North America, Roger T. Peterson and Margaret McKenny. Houghton Mifflin.

(This last book is organized by color and is therefore helpful in identifying completely unknown plants.)

49. RULES FOR COLLECTING HERBS

Never collect herbs when they are wet, as the slightest dew, snow or frost will make the plant moldy.

Use only perfect, unfaded, unblemished, insect-free leaves or flowers. Discard all others, as well as any thick wood stems, since they have no value. Use only unblemished roots or bark.

Gather the plant when it is in full bloom, the seed when it is ripening, the bark when it is rising. Dig roots in spring or late autumn and collect barks in spring or autumn.

50. RULES FOR DRYING HERBS

Many country people collect their herbs when they are already dried on the plant. This lessens the strength and medicinal value of the herb, although it can still be used.

Scentless herbs can be dried in the sun, but herbs with an aroma should be entirely dried in the shade, after which they can be put in the sun for a short time to prevent fungus formation. In a cold climate, it is sometimes necessary to use heat because of the possibility of mildew. Use only slow heat.

Roots should be dried in the shade. Slice or put in bunches and store in a cool, dry, airy place.

Barks can be dried in sunlight, except wild cherry bark.

Leaves and flowers should be dried in an airy, dry place, either hung up in medium-sized bunches, or on wire mesh frames; or on shelves or tables under white shelving paper, in which case they should be turned frequently.

DRYING AND STORING HERBS

	Whole Plant	Bark	Flowers	Leaves	Roots
In sun	Can be picked after drying – American Indians and gypsies did this, but it lessened strength of herb.	Dry in sun. Except wild cherry bark.	Best to dry in airy dry place out of sun except for short time. Sun depletes strength of herb. No scented flowers can be dried in sun.	Best to dry in airy dry place out of sun except for short time. Although sun lessens strength of herb, unscented leaves can be dried in the sun.	
In shade			Flowers with aroma must be dried in the shade. Place in sun for short time to prevent fungus.	Leaves with aroma must be dried in shade. Put in sun for short time to prevent fungus.	Dry roots in shade.
Extra heat			Sometimes in cold climate it is necessary to use extra heat because of possibility of mildew. Use *slow* gas or electric heat only.		
Storage			Dry in medium bunches and hang in dry air, or place on wire mesh frames, or under white shelving paper, or on long tables and turn often.	Dry in medium bunches and hang in dry air, or place on wire mesh frames, or under white shelving paper, or on long tables and turn often.	Store in cool dry airy place.

SOURCES

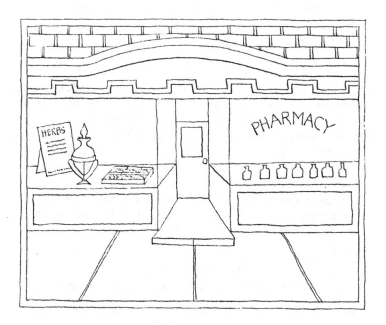

Here is an extensive list of suppliers for herbs, herbal products, books on herbs, and also specialized products for children, organic foods and other products I consider as being valuable for promoting and enhancing health. I've also listed herbal societies and professional organizations for those who are interested in more intense exploration of this fascinating area.

These are volatile times for the economy, and businesses do

move about or even, alas, pass from the scene, so the information here, accurate when I gathered it, is subject to change by the time you read it.

SOURCES FOR MISCELLANEOUS HERBAL PRODUCTS

There are many effective herbal medicine and beauty products on the market. Here are some that may prove valuable to you and your family.

Allergy Products

Eclectic Institute, a Portland, Oregon company, produces freeze-dried stinging nettle capsules which are available in better health stores. To use: At first evidence of an allergic attack, take one to two capsules every other hour as needed. Before season: take bioflavonoids, especially quercetin, which can be combined with vitamin C, and continue dosage of 400 mg twice a day between meals until the end of the allergy season.

Bioforce makes a homeopathic product, Pollinosan, for the relief of symptoms associated with hay fever and similar allergies. There are other excellent homeopathic remedies for allergies.

Analgesic Products
(for relief of pain, arthritis and neuralgia, muscles)

Arnica liniment, ointment (external on unbroken skin) and pills (internal) are first choice for most muscle aches and pains. Health stores and mail order. Tiger Balm is another excellent external herbal ointment for aches and pains. Health stores and drug stores. Haussmann's Pharmacy in Philadelphia carries several homeopathic ointments. Health stores carry Nature's Herbs Boswellin Cream, an Ayurvedic herbal ointment that includes potent capsaicin (extract of cayenne or red pepper). Drug stores stock a Parke-Davis ointment, Zostrix, an over-the-counter product which also is made of capsaicin. It helps with nerve-end pain such as shingles. Carpal tunnel, burns (even radiation burns), and tennis elbow pain respond to pure aloe potions. Aloe Flex is a Texas company that grows its own aloe, 1-800-231-0839, and has effectual aloe ointments. For premium quality aloe leaves: Aloe King, P.O. Box 8335, Saddle Brook, NJ 07662

Castor oil is an extraordinary product for topical healing compresses of chronic pain. Buy in health store or mail order through Heritage Store, 1-800-726-2232, P.O. Box 44-U, Virginia Beach, VA 23458. Heritage also carries pure body and massage oils and natural medicines. The Swiss company Olbas makes analgesic oils, ointments and lotions as well as a massage oil and inhalants for sinus problems. Available through health stores and Penn Herb Co., Ltd., Philadelphia, PA 19123. 1-800-523-9771 for catalog.

Antiseptic Products

Tea Tree Oil, which is distilled from the leaves of Australia's *Melaleuc alternifolia* tree, is a natural antiseptic and antifungal originally used by the Aborigines of Australia. It is available in oil, tincture or capsule form as well as in some toothpastes, breath fresheners, throat lozenges. If not in local health stores: Thursday Plantation, Inc., 118 Nopalitos Way, Santa Barbara, CA 93103. 1-800-848-8966.

Colds, Cough, Flu Products

A wide variety of herbs help abort colds, coughs and flu. Here are some *products* which will prove valuable: Dr. Singha's Mustard Bath is useful to soothe and purify the body, and prevent and overcome a cold. Natural Therapeutics, 2500 Side Cove, Austin, TX 78704 1-800-856-2862. Boiron's homeopathic remedy Oscillococcinum will abort an oncoming flu attack if used at the first sign of symptoms of fever, chills, body aches and pains. Available through several mail order catalogs and from local health stores. Thayer of Concord, MA 01742, has been making Slippery Elm lozenges for over a century and a half. Use them to soothe an irritated throat. The Swiss company, Ricola makes excellent herbal lozenges and "pearls" to soothe an irritated throat. The lozenges are found in health stores and some drug stores.

Detoxification Baths

Hayflower Bath Extract. The Swiss Company, Biokosma makes this extraordinary bath from pure alpine flowers plus horse chestnut and juniper. Use in small amounts for a potent detoxification experience. Available through health stores or mail order from the oldest pharmacy in the United States: Caswell-Massey. Call 1-800-326-0500 for catalog.

Abra 1-800-745-0761 makes a cellular detoxification bath, and a stress therapy bath. Call number for name and number of nearest health store or distributor.

Digestive Aid

Many herbs act as carminatives. Melisana is an invaluable digestive aid. Available only in Europe. M.C.M. Klosterfrau, D 5000 Cologne 1, Germany makes this ancient convent recipe.

Ginger Wonder Syrup from New Moon extracts, Brattleboro, VT, 1-800-543-7279. The syrup is made with freshly extracted organic ginger root and Vermont honey. Use as a short cut for making ginger tonic, or ginger ale. Available in health stores.

Neck Pillow

Hand Picked Products, 75 Van Buren St., San Francisco, CA 94131, 1-800-998-0695, sells these Japanese-style buckwheat hull neck pillows

Medicinal Teas

Hundreds of herbs are useful for medicinal purposes. If you prefer combinations of herbs, Strato Enterprises, Inc., 7 Woodruff Rd. Edison, NJ 08820, (908) 549-4677, sells medicinal teas developed in Germany for a variety of health problems.

Memory Aid

Ginkgo (herb) in capsules, sometimes with choline, can help with memory and alertness as well as circulation. It is said to help in ringing of the ears (tinnitus).

Skin Aids

The Body Shop, 1-800-541-2535 for excellent catalog of wide-ranging natural body products, exfoliants, lotions, soaps, bath oils
Caswell-Massey, 1-800-326-0500. Interesting catalog of world-wide skin, hair, body products
Dr. Hauschka Skin Care Preparations, 1-800-247-9907 are available in many health stores. The products use fresh herbs grown in bio-dynamic gardens.
Herbal Citrus Fruit Exfoliant (Paul Penders) In health stores or call 1-800-4-PENDERS (736-3377) for information
Silica Gel comes from Nature Works, Agoura Hills, CA 91301. This is a mineral supplement for healthy skin, hair and nails. Available in health stores.
Summit Botanicals, P.O. Box 9736, Denver, CO 80209 manufactures Desert Products, natural hair, skin, bath and sun protection products made with extremes of Arizona desert (or any other dry areas) in mind.

Tonics

Norfolk Punch, a Benedictine monk's non-alcoholic herbal tonic. In some health stores or write Norfolk Punch, Welle Manor, Upwell, Norfolk, England PE149AB
Swedish Bitters, a multi-herb tonic and restorative. Available from health stores or write Nature Works, Inc. Agoura Hills, CA 91301

MAIL ORDER: CALL OR WRITE FOR CATALOG

Herbs: Organic

ABRA
Forestville, Ca
1-800-745-0761

Warren Raysor, the dedicated hydrotherapist and herbalist behind ABRA (and Abracadabra) is an authority on herbal therapeutic baths. His products include an excellent cellular detox bath, a stress therapy bath, and sleep bath. He sells only through distributors, so call the number to find out the nearest distributor or store in your area

Blake's Natural Herbs and Spices
505 N. Railroad
Ellensburg, WA 98926
1-800 932-HERB
Organic and nonradiated herbs and spices

Blessed Herbs
Route 5, Box 1042
Ava, MO 65608
(417) 683-5721
Wildcrafted and organic dried herbs

Dry Creek Herb Farm
13035 Dry Creek Rd.
Auburn, CA 95602
(916) 878-2441
Organically grown herbs

Great Lakes Herb Company
P.O. Box 6713
Minneapolis, MN 55406
Organic herbs, bath products. $1.00 catalog

Terra Firma Botanicals, Inc,
126 Sutherlin Lane
Eugene, OR 95405
Wildcrafted and organic herbal products, fresh and dried herbal extracts, flower oils, skin salves, massage oils. $1.00 catalog. Refundable with first order.

Herbs: Miscellaneous

Aphrodisia
264 Bleecker Street
New York, NY 10014
(212) 989-6440
Dried herbs, potpourri, books

Earth's Essence
28 Chester Turnpike,
Auburn, NH 03032
$2.00 catalog. 100 herbal products, bath oils, flower essences, skin and hair care, detoxification products, books and videos

Gaia Botanicals
Box 8485
Philadelphia, PA 19101
$5.00 check or money order for 100 page catalog, or write for free information. 800 herbs, spices including Chinese, Ayurvedic, books, videos

R. Hartenthaler
133 Henderson
Norwood, PA 19074
Bulk medicinal and culinary herbs, green tea, essential oils, herbal combinations, books. $1.00 for catalog, refunded with first order

Harney & Sons, Ltd
Salisbury, CT 06068
1-800-TEA TIME (832-8463)

If you like teas you should make the acquaintance of the Harney clan. John Harney is a master tea blender who learned the art from the British. In the past few years they have blended non-caffeine, *herbal* teas so favored for the table in Europe: tilleul (linden), lemon verbena, or vervaine. The Harney's make a strong chamomile tea that contains only *flower heads*. They also have peppermint, raspberry, lemon, and chunky, flavorful teas made from dried fruits.

Harvest Health, Inc.
1944 Eastern Ave.
S.E. Grand Rapids, MI 49507
(616) 245-6268

Bulk herbs and spices

Haussmann's Pharmacy
534 West Girard Avenue
Philadelphia, PA 19123
1-800 235-5522

herbs by the pound, in capsules, homeopathic products, potpourri.

Health Center For Better Living
6189 Taylor Rd.
Naples, FL 33942-1823
(813) 566-2611 Fax (813) 566-9508

A wide variety of medicinal herbs in 8 forms: whole, ground, powder, tea bags, cut and sifted, granules, flowers, capsules

(The) Herb and Spice Collection
P.O. Box 118
Norway, Iowa 52318
1-800 786-1388

160-page herbal mail order catalog listing 5,000 products. $2.00, refundable first order.

Homestead Herbs
2223 Cold Springs Lane
Spring Garden, CA 95971
    Dream pillows, sachets, potpourri, herbs, spices, teas

Indiana Botanic Gardens Herbalist Catalog.
P.O. Box 5
Hammond, IN 46325
(219) 947-4040
    Herbal products.

Just for the Fun of It
P.O. Box 1521
Lakeport, CA 95453
1-800 601-HERB (4372)

Quakertown Naturals
(818) 968-2736
    Herbs, natural cosmetics, homeopathy, books, herbs and other
healthy foods for the body

Sierra
P.O. Box 412
Kinderhook, NY 12106
1-800 695-2349
    Herbal products, homeopathic remedies

Tatra Herb Company
P.O. Box 60
Morrisville, PA 19067
(215) 295-5476
Herbs, books, remedies, oils. Free catalog

White Crane Trading Co.
447 10th Avenue
New York, NY 10001
(212) 736-1467
FAX (201) 656-3665
    Herbs (ginseng, goldenseal, echinacea, etc.), herbal products
and seeds

Wild Weeds
P.O.Box 88
Redway, CA 95560
(707) 943-3835
Dried herbs and herbal products

Tinctures

A wide variety of medicinal and cosmetic aid tinctures are available in better health stores. Most herbs are extracted in alcohol and are safe to use in this form.

For **nonalcoholic** tinctures check stores for products marked nonalcoholic. One source: Nature's Answer 1-800-645-5720 offers product information and location of nearby seller.

Essential Oils

Organic

Inner Essence
212 E Crest Drive,
Eugene, OR 97405
1-800 821-3029
Organic essential oils and bodycare products.

Miscellaneous Oils

Aroma Vera
5901 Rodeo Rd.
Los Angeles, CA 90016
1-800 669-9514

(The) Good Earth Store,
P.O. Box 129
Liverpool, NY 13088
Sample and catalog, $2.00. Essential oils, massage oils and natural products for body. Custom blending available

Simplers Botanical
P.O. Box 39
Forestville, CA 95436
(707) 887-2012

So Precious,
P.O.Box 3623C,
Long Beach, CA 90803

Uncommon Scents,
P.O.Box 1941
1-800 426-4336
  Custom-scented body care products.

Also refer to these other listings: Body Shop, Caswell-Massey
Co., Ltd., Earth's Essence, R. Hartenthaler, Haussman Pharmacy,
Herb and Spice Collection, Tatra Herb Co., Terra Firma
Botanicals.

Herbs for Children

Weleda,Inc.
P.O.Box 769
Spring Valley, NY 10977
1-800 241-1030 for catalog.
(914) 268-8572

Medicines and body care products from Weleda are based on
the anthroposophical principles of Rudolf Steiner. The renowned
children's products: baby oil, soap and cream are made of organic
calendula. Weleda products, including adult products such as arnica massage oil, chamomile extract, body lotions and mouth products are available in the better health stores.

Herbs For Kids
Box 837
Bozeman, MT 59771
1-800 735-0299
  Organic, alcohol-free, sweet-tasting herb tinctures for the common maladies of childhood. Available in better health stores.

Aromasaurus Rex
Abracadabra
Forestville, CA 95436
1-800-745-0761
  Safe, sudsing biodegradable, nontoxic aromatherapy bath for nonstop children. Contains minute amounts of calming valerian.

Tonics

A. Wolman Formulations
136 SW Washington
Corvallis, OR 97333
(503) 758-8244
  Nonalcohol, nonglycerin herbal memory and brain toner extract

Mrs. Song's Herbal Tonic Soups
The Very Good Soup Company
379a Clementina St.
San Francisco, CA 94103
(415) 441-5505
Fax (415) 243-0194
  Chinese tonic herbs in dry soup mixes

Roots and Legends
38 Miller Avenue
Mill Valley, CA 94941
(415) 381-5631
  Chinese tonic soups, teas and elixirs. $1.00 for catalog, refundable with order

Mail Order Culinary, Cosmetic, Medicinal Herb Plants

Capriland Herb Farm
Silver Street
Coventry,CT 06238
(203) 742-7244
　Herb seeds and plants, dried herbs, potpourri

Cricket Hill Herb Farm, Ltd.
Glen Street
Rowley, MA 01969
(508) 948-2818
　Seeds and plants

Elixir Farm Botanicals
General Delivery
Brixey, MO 65618
　Catalog $2.00. Chinese and indigenous medicinal plant seeds

Fox Hill Farm
443 West Michigan Avenue
P.O. Box 9
Parma, MI 49269
(517) 531-3179

Hartman's Herb Farm
Old Dana Road
Barre, MA 01005
(508) 355-2015
　Seeds and plants.

Nichols Garden Nursery
1190 North Pacific Highway
Albany, OR 97321
　Besides selling peppermint oil straight from the peppermint
fields of Oregon, Nichols sells a long list of hard-to-find herb

plants, gardening supplies, herbal books. Shipping of herb plants start April 1 and continues to June 15.

The Sandy Mush Herb Nursery
316 Surrett Cove Road
Leicester, NC 28748-9622
   Handbook/catalog, mainly culinary, fragrant, some unusual herbs, seeds, herb books, garden books. $4.00, deductible from order.

St. John's Herb Garden, Inc.
7711 Hillmeade Road
Bowie, MD 20720
(301) 262-5302
   Seeds and plants.

Stillridge Herb Farm
10370 Route 99
Woodstock, MD 21163
(301) 465-8348

The Tool Shed Farm
Salem Center
Purdy's Station, NY 10578
1-800 678-7301
   Plants.

Well Sweep Herb Farm
317 Mount Bethel Road
Port Murray, NJ 07865
(201) 852-5390
   Seeds and plants.

TOLL-FREE 800 NUMBERS FOR
MAIL ORDER PURCHASES

Abra, Abracadabra   1-800-745-0761
Allergy Resources   1-800 USE FLAX (872-3529)
Aloe Flex Products   1-800-231-0839
Aroma Vera   1-800- 669-9514

Blake's Natural Herbs and Spices   1-800-932-HERB (4372)
BodyLift   1-800- 443-3917
Body Shop   1-800-541-2535

CamoCare   1-800-CAMOCARE (226-6273)
Caswell-Massey   1-800-326-0500

Diamond Organics   1-800-922-2396
Diet K   1-800-367-5433
Dr. Hauschka Skin Care Products   1-800-247-9907

Ecology Box   1-800-735-1371

FleaBusters, Inc.   1-800-666-3532

Ginger Wonder Syrup   1-800-540-7279

Hand Picked Products   1-800-998-0695
Haussmann Pharmacy   1-800-235-5522
Herbs for Kids   1-800-735-0299
Herb and Spice Collection   1-800-786-1388
Heritage Store   1-800-726-2232

Inner Essence   1-800-821-3029

Just for the Fun of It   1-800-601-HERB (4372)

Morrills' New Directions   1-800-368-5057
(Dr. Singha's) Mustard Bath   1-800-856-2862

Nature's Answer   1-800-645-5720
NuBrush   1-800-NUBRUSH (682-7874)

Paul Penders Herbal Citrus Exfoliant   1-800-4-PENDERS (473-6337)
Penn Herb (Olbas)   1-800-523-9771

Reviva Labs   1-800-257-7774

Self Care Catalog   1-800-345-3371
Seventh Generation   1-800-456-1139
Shitaki Mushrooms   1-800-372-0400
Shivani   1-800-BEST 221 (237-8221)
Sierra   1-800-695-2349
Simmons Holistics   1-800-533-6779

Tool Shed Farm   1-800-678-7301
Tucson Cooperative Warehouse   1-800-350-2667

Uncommon Scents   1-800-426-4336

Vitamin Shoppe   1-800-223-1216

Walnut Acres   1-800-433-3998
Weleda   1-800-726-2232
Wellness Products   1-800-935-5776

HERBAL BOOKS

Harvest Harmony
P.O. Box 1265
McAfree, NJ 07428
(201) 764-4494

Bastyr Books
144 N.E. 154th Street
Seattle, WA 98105
(206) 523-9585 ext 105

Woman of Wands
P.O. Box 330 (Main Street)
South Lee, MA 01260
(213) 243-4036

Also check these resources: Aphrodisia, Earth's Essence, Gaia Botanicals, R. Hartenthaler, Quaker Naturals. Samuel Weiser, New York, also carries a huge list of health and herbal books.

HERBAL AND NATURAL PET RESOURCES

The health of your pet can impact on your health.

American Holistic Veterinary Medical Association
2214 Old Emmorton Rd.
Bel Air, MD 21015
(410) 569-0795
Why is your dog so allergic to flea bites? A holistic practitioner will inquire into food and environmental allergies, vaccines, genetic disposition and possible immune dysfunction.
For a list of local practitioners, send a large stamped, self-self-addressed envelope.

Morrills' New Directions
P.O. Box 30
Orient, ME 04471
1-800 368-5057
Natural pet care catalog including herbs, vitamins and books, natural wormers, homeopathic remedies and herbal remedies for summer pest problems. $1.00 for catalog, refundable with order.

Natural Pet Products
1888 Century Park East, 19th Floor
Los Angeles, CA 90067
(310) 284-3161
NPP sells flea powder, collars, sprays and shampoos.

FleaBusters, Inc
N.W. Ninth Ave. #411
Ft. Lauderdale, Fl 33309
1-800-666-3532
A nonpesticide flea product for the home.

Williams Industries
P.O. Box 7203
Rocky Mount, NC 27804
(919) 442-3160
The Williams flea trap to capture fleas. Available in hardware
and pet stores.

To repel fleas: Use garlic tablets and yeast in pet food. Prepare
this 16 ounce spray: 1 cup of water, 2 tablespoons apple cider
vinegar, 1 cup Avon's Skin-So-Soft. Apply onto coat with fingers
every few days.

Allergy to cats? The primary cat allergen deposited on carpets
and upholstery can be controlled with a homemade herbal spray
made of water and 3% tannic acid: (herb) oak bark, coffee, cocoa
and tea. See Vol. 138, no 7 *Science News*: investigation of Aller-
gist Jeffery Miller, Danbury, Conn., and researcher Thomas A.E.
Platts-Mills of University of Virginia, Charlottesville.

HERBAL HEALTH PRACTITIONERS

Contact these organizations for referrals to specialized health
practioners. Send large stamped, self-addressed envelope (SSAE)
for information.

American Herbalists Guild
P.O. Box 1683
Soquel, CA 95073
(408) 464-2441

American Association of Naturopathic Physicians
2366 Eastlake Ave. E., Suite 322
Seattle, WA 98102

National Association for Holistic Aromatherapy
3072 Edison Ct.
Boulder, CO 80301
(303) 444-0533

HERBAL SOCIETIES AND ASSOCIATIONS

USA

American Herbal Products Association
P.O. Box 2410
Austin, TX 78768
(512)320-8555
Fax (512)320-8908

American Botanical Council
Box 201660
Austin, TX 78720
(512) 331-8868

Herb Research Foundation
1007 Pearl Street, Suite 200
Boulder, CO 80302
1-800-748-2617

The International Herb Growers and Marketers Association
P.O.Box 281
Silver Spring, PA 17575
(717) 285 4252

Great Britain

The British Herb Trade Association, c/o Administrator
NFU House
London SWIX7NJm
071-235-5077
Fax 071 235-3526

The Herb Society
P.O. Box 559
London SW114RW
0296 625126

The British Herbal Medicine Association
Field House
Lye Hole Lane
Redhill, Avon BS1871B

The British Homeoepathic Association
27a Devonshire Street
London WIN1RJ

Henry Doubleday Research Association
Ryton Gardens
National Centre for Organic Gardening
Ryton-on-Dunsmore, Coventry CV83LG

The National Institute of Medicinal Herbalists
9 Palace Gate
Exeter EX11JA

The Royal Horticultural Society
Vincent Square
London
SW1P2PE

Australia

The Academy of Natural Healing Pty Ltd
7 The Esplanade
Ashfield, New South Wales
Australia 2131

The Herb Society of South Australia
P.O. Box 140
Parkside, S. Australia 5063

National Herbalists Association of Australia (Queensland Chapter)
Montville Road
Mapleton, Queensland
Australia 4560

The Queensland Herb Society
23 Greenmount Avenue
Holland Park, Brisbane, Queensland
Australia

The Tasmanian Herb Society
12 Delta Avenue
Tarrona, Tasmania 7006

New Zealand

The Auckland Herb Society
P.O. Box 20022
Glen Eden, Auckland 7
New Zealand

South Africa

The Herb Society of South Africa
PO Box 5783
Durban, Republic of South Africa

HEALTH AND ENVIRONMENT CATALOGS

Self-Care and Diagnostic Tests

Self Care Catalog
5850 Shellmound
Emeryville, CA 94608
1-800-345-3371 or (510) 658-0970
   Some herb products, but mostly exceptional self-care and fitness products, and home diagnostic tests including blood pressure monitors, bladder infection tests, colorectal cancer screening test, home pregnancy tests

   American Diabetes Association (local) or national at (703) 549-1500 for home blood glucose monitor buyer's guide

Environment

Seventh Generation
49 Hercules Dr.
Colchester, VT 05446-1672
1-800-456-1139
   Environmentally safe home, health, self-care products

The Ecology Box
2260 S. Main St.
Ann Arbor, MI 48103
1-800-735-1371

The Natural Choice
Eco Design Company
1365 Tufina Circle
Santa Fe, NM 87501
   Information: (505) 438-3448, Orders: 1-800-621-2591, Fax: (505) 438-0199
   Everything from natural bedding to a natural shower curtain and

house paints. They carry organic marigold shampoo, and a nettles and rosemary as well as Moroccan volcanic clay shampoo, soap and oil spa stones, and an eastern sea bodybrush (Rikko) for use in the bath.

Tucson Cooperative Warehouse
350 South Toole Avenue,
Tucson, AZ 85701
1-800-350-2667
Fax (602) 792-3258
　Health and environmental products. Herbal teas and 4500 natural foods and Earth-friendly nonfood products. Coop with deliveries to six nearby states, and mail order elsewhere. They will help you to start a buying club in your area.

Lighting

Walnut Acres
1-800-433-3998
Special Daylight-corrected bulbs

Simmons Holistics
P.O. Box 3193
Chattanooga, TN 37404
1-800-533-6779
　Full-spectrum lights helpful in seasonal affective disorder, and incandescent chromalux color-corrected bulbs

Wellness Products
P.O. Box 40374
St. Petersburgh, FL 33743
1-800-935-5776
　Antiradiation desk lamp

Allergy

NuBrush
Applied Microdontics, Inc.
24681 La Plaza, Suite 310
Dana Point, CA 92629
1-800-NUBRUSH (682-7874)
   Antibacterial toothbrush spray

Allergy Resources
P.O. Box 888
Palmer Lake, CO 80133
1-800-USE FLAX (872-3529)
   Products for a healthier lifestyle.

Anti-Gravity Stand

BODYLIFT
P.O. Box 1667
Newport Beach, CA 92663
1-800-443-3917
   An easy yoga headstand aid

Miscellaneous

Cutting Edge Catalog
Befit Enterprises Ltd.
P.O. Box 2143
Southampton, NY 11969

HOMEOPATHIC SOURCES

Local health stores and pharmacies

Haussmann's Pharmacy   1-800-235-5522
Quakertown Naturals   (818) 968-2736
Sierra   1-800-695-2349

Seeds of Nature
P.O. Box 2144
Great Neck, NY 11020
(516) 482-8719
Fax (516) 482-4320
Complete homeopathic guide for better health

Vitamin Shoppe catalog   1-800-223-1216

ORGANIC FOODS BY MAIL

Walnut Acres
Penns Creek, PA 17862
1-800-433-3998
This organic farm was started in 1946 and is still going strong under the Keene family. Fresh, certified organic foods canned from the field. Complete array of certified products for the table and herbal products, vegetable washes, natural insect repellents, and a complete line of full-spectrum lights, incandescent and fluorescent, to satisfy your craving for natural sunlight and daylight.

Diamond Organics
Freedom, CA 95019
1-800-922-2396
Organically grown fruits and vegetables available the year round to U.S. and Canada

Jaffe Bros.
Valley Center, CA 92082-0636
Save on bulk buying organic and other natural foods. In business for 45 years.

MISCELLANEOUS FOOD

Shiitaki Mushrooms Vermont Forrest Farm
W. Topsham, VT 05086
1-800-372-0400
An excellent mail-order source for immune-building mushrooms imported from Japan. Sold by the pound, plus shipping. Visa, MasterCard.

BOTANICAL, PHARMACEUTICAL, FOOD USAGE CHART

Herb	Skin	Hair	Eyes	Mouth	Feet
Almond meal	facial roughness, dryness, wrinkles, blackheads				
Almond oil	lotion	conditioner, growth			
Alum	tightener	darken hair			
Angelica					
Anise					
Apple	dryness, pimples			mouthwash	
Apricot	facial, vitamin A				
Artichoke		darken hair, growth			
Avocado	facial dryness, nourishment, cleanser	conditioner, shampoo			
Bay					
Balsam of Gilead	circulation, tightener, wrinkles, facial				
Barley	facial wrinkles, pimples				
Bay leaf					
Bayberry 1) bark 2) root				X	
Bentonite	facial thickener, healing				

Nails	Hands	Deodorant	Bath	Sleep	Astringent	Miscel-laneous
	lotion					scrub, external
	aid					
				pillow		
				tablets		
				X		
						external
						external
	conditioner					external
						aroma
						external
						scrub, external
					X	
					X	

Herb	Skin	Hair	Eyes	Mouth	Feet
Benzoin	tightener, circulation, wrinkles, blemishes, cleaner				
Bindweed					swollen feet
Biotin		growth			
Birch sap	blemishes				
Bistort root				tooth powder	
Blackberry leaf					
Black cohosh					
Blackstrap molasses		growth, internal			
Borax	bleach, softener				
Boric acid powder			X		powder
Bouncing bet (soapwort)					
Boxwood shavings		X			
Bran	facial, large pores, dryness, tightening				
Brandy	oiliness, chap, roughness	oiliness			
Brewer's yeast	acne, pimples, eczema, oiliness, dryness, secretions of the skin, facial	problems		creases	

Nails	Hands	Deodorant	Bath	Sleep	Astringent	Miscel-laneous
						aroma fixative, simple tincture
						internal
						internal
					X	
			X external			menstrua-tion, internal
				X		internal
	cream		softener			external
						soap
		internal				cleanse, external
			scrub			external
	lotion					external
split nails, hangnails		internal				internal, external

Herb	Skin	Hair	Eyes	Mouth	Feet
Burdock root	acne				
Buttermilk	facial, bleaching, tightening, large pores, sunburn, oiliness				
Cactus					
Calamus root					
Calcium		external			
Camphor (gum)	facial, tightener, soothing, large pores	reviver		toothpaste	
Carbonate of soda					
Carnation					
Carrot	facial, pimples, vitamin A				
Cassia bud					
Castor oil	liver, age spots	strength-ener, con-ditioner, reviver			
Catechu		hair dye			
Catnip		dandruff, external			swelling, internal
Cat's tail	blemishes				swelling, internal
Cayenne pepper				gargle	powder for warmth
Celandine			X	X	

Nails	Hands	Deodorant	Bath	Sleep	Astringent	Miscellaneous
						cleanser, internal
						external
				internal		
						potpourri
aid, internal				tablets, internal		
		internal				
			stimulating			external
						aroma
						internal, external
						aroma
						external

Herb	Skin	Hair	Eyes	Mouth	Feet
Celery	pimples		X		
Chamomile	facial, wrinkles, soothing, external	blond rinse, blond dye	compress, soothes puffiness		
Chickweed	freckles				
Chicory			strength-ener		
Chlorogalum	soap	shampoo			
Chrysan-themum					
Cinnamon					
Cleavers					
Clove		growth, external		mouthwash	
Cocoa butter	facial, creams, stretch marks	conditioner			
Coconut		shampoo			
Collard greens	internal				
Coltsfoot	veins				
Comfrey	facial, healing wrinkles, regenerates new cells		cream		
Cornmeal	cleanser, facial, large pores, soother, scrub				
Costmary					
Couch grass	blemish				swelling

Nails	Hands	Deodorant	Bath	Sleep	Astringent	Miscellaneous
						internal
			soothing, external	tea, internal	X	insect bites, external
			X			external
						internal
		X				
				X		potpourri
		X				
				internal		aroma
	lotion					
	healing					
			body cleanser			external
						aroma
						internal

Herb	Skin	Hair	Eyes	Mouth	Feet
Cowslip (English)	whitener, wrinkles				
Cramp bark					leg cramps
Cranberry juice	moles, external				
Cresses	salve, blemishes				
Cuckoopint	blemishes, cleanser				
Cucumber	cooling, tightening, nourishing, large pores, oiliness		soothing		
Daisy	pimples, blotches				
Damiana					
Dandelion	internal				
Dogwood twig				toothbrush, tooth whitener	
Egg white	facial tightener, large pores, wrinkles, pimples, puffiness, sunburn, oiliness				
Egg yolk	facial, dry skin, conditioner	conditioner			
Elder 1) berry		black dye			X

Nails	Hands	Deodorant	Bath	Sleep	Astringent	Miscel-laneous
						cleanser
						internal
				internal		
					pore tightener	external
				X		
					pore tightener	external
	X					external

Herb	Skin	Hair	Eyes	Mouth	Feet
Elder 2) flower	facial, complexion waters, bleach, wrinkles, blemishes		healer		
3) leaf					powder
Endive			internal		
Epsom salt	double chin bandage, blackheads				
Escarole			strengthener		
Eucalyptus					
Eyebright			wash, in-flammation, puffiness		
Fennel	facial wrin-kles, impurities		compress		
Fern					foot bath, cures fatigue, leg cramps
Fig			X		
Flaxseed (linseed)	softener in facial	setting lotion	compress		
Folic acid		internal			
Fuller's earth	thickener for facial	dry shampoo			
Garlic					corn

Nails	Hands	Deodorant	Bath	Sleep	Astringent	Miscellaneous
			curative, stimulating, soothing	X		external
			curative, relieves aches			external
						internal
			curative, body aches			
						internal, external
			curative			external
						constipation
barrier, protective cream						

Herb	Skin	Hair	Eyes	Mouth	Feet
Gelatine	thickener for facial	setting lotion, gives body			
Geranium					swelling
Gladwin	sores, itches, scabs				
Glycerine	facial, moisturizing emollient, double chin bandage, healing				
Goldenrod					
Goldensea	healer		compress		X
Grape	dry skin, tan, sunburn, freckles, external				
Grapefruit					
Gum arabic	tightener	setting lotion			
Gum tragacanth	facial tightener, large pores			X	
Hay flower	curative				problems
Heliotrope					
Henna		hair dye			
Holm oak		darken hair			
Honey	facial, healing, mois- turizing, wrinkles, blackheads, large pores, nourishing, external	blond dye			

Nails	Hands	Deodorant	Bath	Sleep	Astringent	Miscellaneous
internal strengthener						
						external
	lotion, healing					
			external			
				internal		
				hot juice		
					X	aroma fixative
					X	aroma fixative, scent balls
			curative			
						aroma
nail dye						
nail aid			nourishing	retains body fluids, internal		with apple cider is reviving, internal

Herb	Skin	Hair	Eyes	Mouth	Feet
Hops					
Horseradish	bleaching (grated), acne (compound spirit)				
Horsetail	facial, large pores, oiliness, internal, external		reduces swelling, external		stimulating, external
Houseleek	facial, wrinkles, healing, nourishing creams				corn
Indian corn	blemishes				swelling
Inositol		anti-grey, aids growth			
Irish moss	softener for facial	setting lotion			
Ivy twig	sunburn				
Jaborandi		growth stimulat- ing			
Jasmine					
Juniper					
Kaolin	thickener in facial	filler for dye			
Karaya Gum	tightner	setting lotion			
Kelp		oilines			

Nails	Hands	Deodorant	Bath	Sleep	Astringent	Miscel-laneous
				tea in pillows		
						external
regener-ates, external			curative, stimulat-ing, external		X	
						external
						internal
			X			aroma
				X		
	protective in cream					
					X	
						use instead of salt

Herb	Skin	Hair	Eyes	Mouth	Feet
Lady's mantle (whole herb)	facial, lotion, creams, acne, wrinkles, inflammation				
Lady's slipper					
Lamb's quarters (pigweed)	cleanser				
Lanolin	facial, creams, moisturizer, emollient, wrinkles				
Laurel		darkens hair			
Lavender water/oil		wash		clean teeth, gargle	cures fatigue
Lecithin	facial, acne				
Lemon	facial, spring cleaner, restores acidity, large pores, oiliness, blackheads, external	setting lotion, external		tooth cleaner, external	
Lemon balm					
Lemon verbena					

Nails	Hands	Deodorant	Bath	Sleep	Astringent	Miscel-laneous
	X		soothing	tea under pillow promotes sleep	very astringent	can flush kidneys, external, internal
				X		
						soap
			liquid			
		external	aroma	pillow		aroma, headache, depression tonic, fever, external
					~	
cuticle aid, external				hot lemonade, internal		
				tea, internal; pillow, external		
				tea, internal; pillow, external		

Herb	Skin	Hair	Eyes	Mouth	Feet
Lettuce, cultivated	eau de laitre, complexion water				
Lettuce, wild					
Lilac flower	cleans, softens				
Lily of the valley					
Lime flower (linden)	facial, wrinkles, large pores, plant hormones, impurities, external				
Linseed (see Flaxseed)					
Liver	pimples	X			
Logwood		darkens hair			
Lovage					
Lupine seed	blemishes, external				
Magnesium		needed			
Maidenhair fern		growth			
Marigold (calendula)	facial, thread veins, healing, wrinkles	red dye	lotion		
Marjoram					
Marshmallow 1) flower 2) root	facial lotion, roughness	hair lightener lotion			

Nails	Hands	Deodorant	Bath	Sleep	Astringent	Miscel-laneous
		internal, external		tea		
				tea		
						use as soap
						aroma
			curative	tea		cleanses system, tranquil-izes, internal
						internal
		external				
						internal
						aroma

Herb	Skin	Hair	Eyes	Mouth	Feet
Melon	dry skin				
Milk	facial, healing, dry skin, rough skin, acne, oiliness, external				
Mint	facial, stimulating, cleansing, external			mouthwash, external	
Mulberry		darken hair			
Mullein		lighten hair			
Mushroom					
Musk					
Myrrh	facial, healing, wrinkles			stimulating to membranes, mouthwash	
Myrtle	blemishes	darken hair			
Narcissus root	facial				
Nettle	facial, cleanser, stimulating, soothing, impurities, plant hormones, external	reviver, dandruff, growth, external	X external	breath sweetener, internal	
Nutmeg		growth		mouthwash	
Oak bark	X				
Oak moss					

Nails	Hands	Deodorant	Bath	Sleep	Astringent	Miscellaneous
			soothing, external	with honey, internal		
			soothing, healing, external			aroma, soothing, cleansing, internal, tea
		internal				
			X			aroma fixative
					X	
						potpourri
	chap chaser					potpourri
		internal	curative		X	
				X		aroma
						scent powder

Herb	Skin	Hair	Eyes	Mouth	Feet
Oat flower	impurities				foot bath problems
Oatmeal	facial, soothing, whitening, blackheads, healing, external				
Olive oil	nourishing, sunburn	nourishing, conditioner			
Onion	blemishes, spots, wrinkles				corn
Orange flower					
Orrisroot		dry shampoo			
PABA	sunburn ointment, external	restorer, growth, internal			
Pantothenic acid		growth, internal			
Papaya	facial, dead skin cleanser external		dark circles, external		
Parsley	facial, thread veins, external	sheen, conditioner, external	compress	breath sweetener, internal	
Parsnip		hair conditioner			
Passion flower					
Patchouli oil					
Patience	pimples				

Nails	Hands	Deodorant	Bath	Sleep	Astringent	Miscellaneous
			curative			
	lotion		soothing, healing, relieves itching			non-allergenic scrub or soap
conditioner						
						external
				tea, internal		aroma
				pillow		fixative, potpourri
		internal				
				X		
		external				aroma

Herb	Skin	Hair	Eyes	Mouth	Feet
Peach 1) fruit 2) leaf	facial moisturizer	reviver, shampoo			
Pellitory of the wall	spots, freckles, pimples, sunburn				
Pennyroyal					
Peppermint	facial, stimulating, tightening, external				
Pimpernel	blemishes, complexion water				
Pineapple juice					
Pine needles					
Plantain (common)	healing		compress		
Plum	X				
Potato	facial, cleansing, nourishing, maintaining, bleach, oiliness, sunburn, external; eczema, internal		puffiness		
Privit		golden dye with radish			
Pulsatilla					

Nails	Hands	Deodorant	Bath	Sleep	Astringent	Miscellaneous
				tea		
				tea, internal; pillow, external		aroma, internal cleanser, calming, soothing
			X			
X						
			eases body aches			
			X			can stop bleeding
				X		

Herb	Skin	Hair	Eyes	Mouth	Feet
Quassia chips		rinse for dark hair, sheen			
Quebracho		darken hair			
Quince seed	softener for facial	growth, setting lotion, golden hair dye			
Radish		golden hair dye			
Raspberry	cleansing, internal			compress	
Red bergamot					
Red clover	skin eruptions				
Red robin (geranium)					reduces swelling, external
Redwood		darken hair			
Restharrow					internal
Rhubarb root		golden hair dye			
Riboflavin	brown spots, internal				
Rose 1) water 2) bud	creams, facial bleaching			mouthwash	
Rose geranium					
Rose hip tea	bleaching freckles		puffiness, dark circles		

Nails	Hands	Deodorant	Bath	Sleep	Astringent	Miscel-laneous
		tops				
			nourisher			menstrual problems, childbirth
				tea		
			X			
	lotion		X			
				in pillows		aroma
						aroma
						internal

Herb	Skin	Hair	Eyes	Mouth	Feet
Rosemary	facial	dandruff, hair wash, setting lotion, reviver, lustre, curls			
Rue (flower)	pimples				
Rum		oily hair, external			
Safflower oil	facial				
Saffron		reddish-blond dye			
Sage	large pores, facial, external	dandruff, darken hair wash		tooth whitener, mouthwash, cleaner	
Salt	invigorating			mouthwash, tooth cleaner	
Sassafras bark	acne		X		
Sesame oil	lotion, suntan facial				
Silver mantle	blemishes				swelling
Silverweed	blemishes, sunburn, pimples, freckles				
Skullcap					
Soapberry					
Southernwood		shampoo, rinse for dark hair			
Soybean		oiliness, internal			

Nails	Hands	Deodorant	Bath	Sleep	Astringent	Miscellaneous
			cleanser, eases body aches	pillows		
				X		
			X			
		controls perspiration	curative	tea, internal; pillow, external		
			before bath body rub			
			X			
						impurities
				tea, internal		
						soap

Herb	Skin	Hair	Eyes	Mouth	Feet
Spike					
Storax					
Strawberry	clears oiliness, internal, external		X	tooth cleaner	
Sulphur water	liver, brown spots, acne, pimples, external				
Sunflower seed and oil	cleanser, nourisher, high in lecithin			strengthens teeth	
Sweet cream	facial, wrinkles, nourishing, external				
Swiss Kriss		darkens hair			
Tag alder root		darkens hair			
Tarragon					
Teasel			X		
Thyme	facial				
Tomato	facial, large pores, nourishing				
Tonquin					
Turkey oil					

Nails	Hands	Deodorant	Bath	Sleep	Astringent	Miscel-laneous
						aroma
						aroma fixative
			X		lotion	
						high in vitamin A, E, calcium, phos-phorus, fluorine
						herbal laxative product
				pillow		
						aroma
					X	
						aroma
			disperses in water			is treated castor oil

Herb	Skin	Hair	Eyes	Mouth	Feet
Turnip top				breath sweetener, internal	
Valerian					
Vervain					
Vetiver					
Vinegar	cleanser, softener, itchiness, flakiness, sunburn, large pores, blackheads, anti-fatigue	dandruff, conditioner, rinse			itchiness
Violet water			compress		
Vitamin A	rough skin, acne, blemishes, infection			gum aid	
Vitamin B complex	dermatitis, dry, scaly	needed		aids receding gums	
Vitamin B$_2$	liver spots				
Vitamin B$_{12}$	eczema				
Vitamin C	infection, black and blue marks			swollen gums, pulp of teeth	leg cramps
Vitamin D					

Nails	Hands	Deodorant	Bath	Sleep	Astringent	Miscellaneous
		internal				
				capsule or tea		
				internal		
		suppresses perspiration				
strengthens			invigorating, lessens fatigue			apple cider preferred
growth						
strengthens		foods containing B are antiperspirant				
ridges						

Herb	Skin	Hair	Eyes	Mouth	Feet
Vitamin E	facial, moisturizer, wrinkles, chin aid, brown liver spots, circulation, internal, external, burns, heals wounds				
Walnut shell		dyes hair darker			
Watercress	blemishes, internal, external				
Wheat germ	facial, thread veins, allergic skin, internal, external				
Wheat germ oil	nourishing, dry skin, chin and neck, allergic skin				
Wild pansy	blemishes				
Willow 1) bark 2) leaves 3) sap	spots dis-colouring	dandruff			bath for weak feet
Wine (white)	blackheads, oiliness, external	wash external			

Nails	Hands	Deodorant	Bath	Sleep	Astringent	Miscel-laneous
						blood cleanser
			recovering illness			

Herb	Skin	Hair	Eyes	Mouth	Feet
Witch hazel	sunburn, puffiness, tightener		puffiness, inflamma- tion, dark circles		
Wood moss					foot bath, leg cramps, fallen arches
Woodruff					
Wormwood	healing, eruptions, scabs, eczema				
Yarrow	facial, dilates pores, cuts grease, internal, external	oiliness			
Yogurt	facial, normal-oily, cleanser, bleach, external				
Yucca	soap	shampoo			

Nails	Hands	Deodorant	Bath	Sleep	Astringent	Miscel-laneous
					pore tightener	
				tea, internal; pillow, external		
					cuts grease	heals wounds, sore nipples

INDEX